Mayo Clinic Guide *to* Integrative Medicine

Published by Time Inc. Books
225 Liberty Street, New York, NY 10281

The information in this book is true and complete to the best of our knowledge. This book is intended only as an informative guide. It is not intended to replace, countermand or conflict with the advice given to you by your physician. Information in this book is offered with no guarantees. The author and publisher disclaim all liability in connection with the use of this book.

For bulk sales to employers, member groups and health-related companies, write Mayo Clinic, 200 First St. SW, Rochester, MN 55905, call 800-430-9699, or email *SpecialSalesMayoBooks@mayo.edu*.

ISBN 13: 978-0-8487-5660-4
Library of Congress Control Number: 2017932106

Printed in the USA
1 2 3 4 5 6 7 8 9 10

In this book we discuss a variety of products and practices. Our intent is for this information to serve as discussion points between the reader and his or her doctor. Because we say a therapy may be beneficial or we give it a "green light" does not mean we are endorsing any specific product or therapy.

IMAGE CREDITS

With the exception of the images on page 203, the individuals pictured in this book are models, and the photos are used for illustrative purposes only. There's no correlation between the individuals portrayed and the condition or subject discussed.

Mayo Clinic

MEDICAL EDITOR
Brent A. Bauer, M.D.

EDITORIAL DIRECTOR
Paula M. Marlow Limbeck

SENIOR EDITOR
Karen R. Wallevand

MANAGING EDITOR
Stephanie K. Vaughan

PRODUCT MANAGER
Christopher C. Frye

ILLUSTRATION, PHOTOGRAPHY AND PRODUCTION
Stewart J. (Jay) Koski, Kent McDaniel, Matthew C. Meyer,
Gunnar T. Soroos, Malgorzata (Gosha) B. Weivoda

EDITORIAL RESEARCH
Abbie Y. Brown, Deirdre A. Herman, Erika A. Riggin

PROOFREADING
Miranda M. Attlesey, Alison K. Baker,
Julie M. Maas

INDEXING
Steve Rath

CONTRIBUTORS
Anjali Bhagra, M.D., Barbara K. Bruce, Ph.D., L.P., Paul
E. Carns, M.D., Tony Y. Chon, M.D., Edward T. Creagan,
M.D., Kevin C. Fleming, M.D., Ralph E. Gay, M.D., D.C.,
Jennifer L. Hauschulz, Jennifer L. Koski, James T Li,
M.D., Ph.D., Connie A. Luedtke, R.N., RN-BC, Denise
M. Millstine, M.D., Arya B. Mohabbat, M.D., Katherine
M. Piderman, Ph.D., Jessica M. Smidt, Amit Sood, M.D.,
Jon C. Tilburt, M.D.

Table of contents

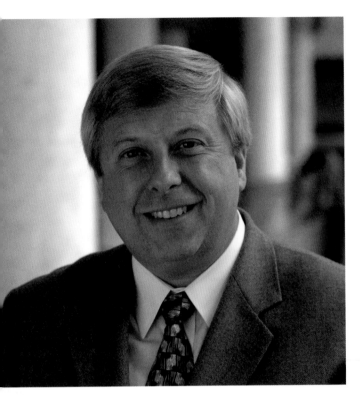

Brent A. Bauer, M.D.
Medical editor, *Mayo Clinic Guide to Integrative Medicine,* and Director of Research, Integrative Medicine and Health, Mayo Clinic, Rochester, Minnesota.

As Americans seek greater control of their health, explosive growth is taking place in the field of integrative medicine. People are looking for more "natural" or "holistic" ways to maintain good health. In addition, more and more people want to not only manage and prevent illness but also improve their quality of life overall.

At the same time, more treatments that were once considered "on the fringe" are slowly being integrated into conventional medicine. The key word to focus on here is "integrated."

Although the term *integrative medicine* may be new to you, it's reflected in the title of this book for a reason. It's a term that's been in the works for many years now — a concept that was known as *alternative medicine* back in 2007 when the *Mayo Clinic Book of Alternative Medicine* was first published. That's because these types of treatments were seen as alternatives to conventional medicine. Since then, the term *alternative medicine* has gone through several evolutions as more is learned about this growing field.

Today, as evidence showing the safety and effectiveness of many of these therapies grows, physicians are starting to integrate aspects of what was once seen as alternative medicine into conventional medical care. That's why you're hearing the term *integrative medicine* more often. That change is reflected in the title of this book.

The purpose behind what you are about to read is to give you evidence-based insight into many of the most popular integrative treatments that can boost your health and wellness. You'll learn about integrative techniques and treatments that Mayo Clinic feels have the best research behind them.

Before you read through this book, think about your current health and your quality of life. If it's not where you want it to be, integrative medicine — used alongside conventional medicine — may be worth discussing with your health care team. What is most important is finding the best evidence-based products and practices that work with conventional medicine to improve your health — mind, body and spirit.

Start your integrative medicine journey

Here are 3 ways you can experience integrative medicine right now, this week.

1. Try one new form of exercise.

Try a different form of physical activity this week. Here are three options.

Yoga
Yoga is a mind-body practice that combines physical poses, controlled breathing, and meditation or relaxation. Before trying yoga, see page 29 to make sure it's safe for you. Find yoga poses to try at *www.MayoClinic.org.* Search on "yoga video."

Tai chi
Tai chi is a self-paced system of gentle physical exercise and stretching. Learn more about tai chi on page 29. Learn how to do tai chi here: *https://nccih.nih.gov/video/taichidvd-full*

Qi gong
Qi gong (CHEE-gung or CHEE-KUNG) generally combines meditation, relaxation, physical movement and breathing exercises to restore and maintain balance. Learn how to practice qi gong here: *https://nccih.nih.gov/video/taichidvd-3*

2. Try a new way to manage your stress this week.

Choose one or more of these techniques:

Progressive muscle relaxation
First, find a quiet place free from interruption. Tense each muscle group for at least five seconds and then relax for up to 30 seconds. Repeat before moving to the next muscle group. Learn more about progressive muscle relaxation on page 44.

Deep breathing
With deep breathing, you breathe from the muscle under your rib cage (diaphragm). Take a deep breath of air, pause, exhale and then pause before repeating. Learn more on page 46.

Guided imagery
Form mental images of places or situations you find relaxing. Use as many senses as possible, such as smells, sights, sounds and textures. Learn more about guided imagery on page 64.

Mindfulness meditation
When you practice mindfulness meditation, focus on what you're experiencing, such as the flow of your breath. Observe your thoughts and emotions, but let them pass without judgment. Learn more about mindfulness meditation on page 57.

3. Do something spiritual for yourself one day this week.

Spirituality can take many different forms:
- Practicing prayer, meditation, deep breathing, expressing gratitude, silent observation, experiencing art and relaxation techniques to help you focus your thoughts.
- Keeping a journal to help you express your feelings and record your progress.
- Seeking out a trusted adviser or friend — someone with similar life experiences — who can help you discover what's important in life.
- Reading inspirational stories or essays to help you evaluate different philosophies in life.
- Connecting with others, such as friends, family or a group that gathers for a spiritual purpose.
- Helping someone in need.
- Reflecting on the bigger picture in life, especially during times of stress.
- Spending time in nature.
- Looking for and doing things that give your life meaning and purpose, such as the work you do or something that helps you feel connected to something larger than yourself.

What is integrative medicine?

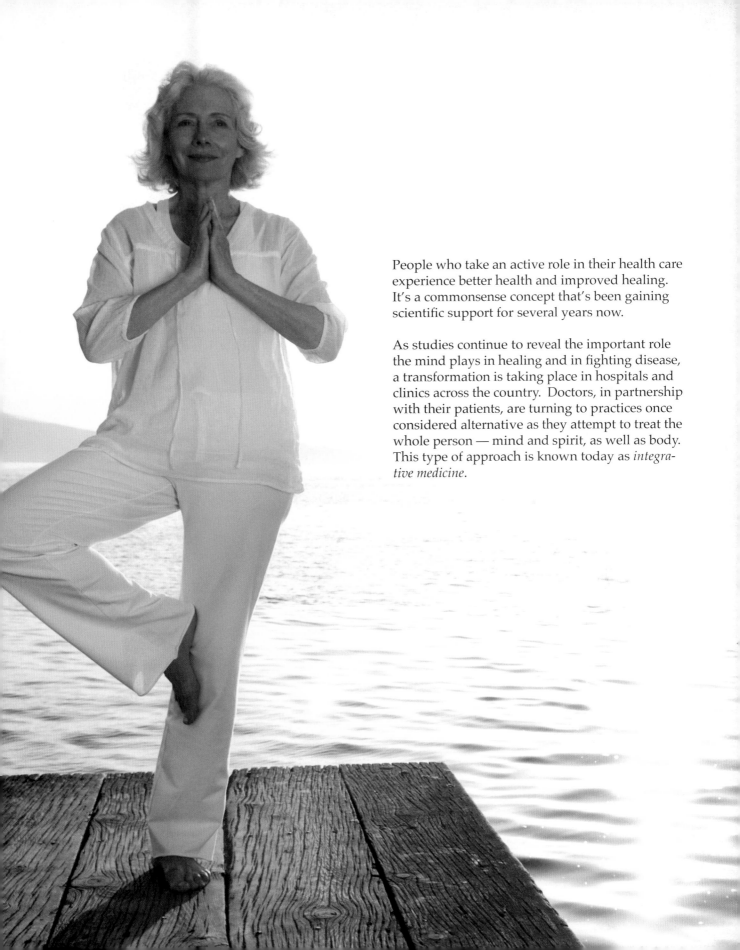

People who take an active role in their health care experience better health and improved healing. It's a commonsense concept that's been gaining scientific support for several years now.

As studies continue to reveal the important role the mind plays in healing and in fighting disease, a transformation is taking place in hospitals and clinics across the country. Doctors, in partnership with their patients, are turning to practices once considered alternative as they attempt to treat the whole person — mind and spirit, as well as body. This type of approach is known today as *integrative medicine*.

What is integrative medicine?

Building a solid wellness foundation means addressing all aspects of your health — mind, body and spirit. The same is true for integrative medicine. As researchers continue to discover the important role the mind plays in healing and in fighting disease, doctors, in partnership with their patients, are turning to practices once considered alternative as they attempt to treat the whole person.

A shift toward wellness

Integrative medicine describes an evolution taking place in many health care institutions. This evolution is due in part to a shift in the medical industry as health care professionals focus on wellness as well as on treating disease. This shift offers a new opportunity for integrative therapies.

Integrative (in-tuh-GRAY-tiv) medicine is the practice of using conventional medicine alongside evidence-based complementary treatments. The idea behind integrative medicine is not to replace conventional medicine, but to find ways to complement existing treatments.

For example, taking a prescribed medication may not be enough to bring your blood pressure level into a healthy range, but adding meditation to your daily wellness routine may give you the boost you need — and prevent you from needing to take a second medication.

Integrative medicine isn't just about fixing things when they're broken; it's about keeping things from breaking in the first place. And in many cases, it means bringing new therapies and approaches to the table, such as meditation, mindfulness and tai chi. Sometimes, integrative approaches help lead people into a complete lifestyle of wellness.

Past and present

Integrative medicine has come a long way in the last 20 years. In the 1990s, integrative medicine started to undergo a major shift. Descriptions such as *unorthodox* or *alternative* were replaced with the term *complementary and alternative medicine* (CAM). CAM, in turn, became an umbrella term for herbal remedies, mind-body therapies, traditional Chinese medicine and more.

Today, as physicians integrate more of these treatments into their medical practices, the term *CAM* has given way to the term *integrative medicine*. As the word *integrative* suggests, integrative medicine describes the integration of natural or holistic practices into the health care paradigm to complement conventional Western medicine and promote wellness.

At first, medical professionals generally disapproved of integrative medicine, which was known at first as "alternative" — meaning an alternative to conventional medicine. Despite this disapproval from the medical establishment, people kept experimenting and trying new approaches to health, often influenced by the medical practices of other cultures.

Why integrative medicine?

Many academic medical centers are taking steps to better understand unconventional treatments and learn about their safety and effectiveness.

To date, over 70 academic medical centers are now part of an organization called the Academic Consortium for Integrative Medicine & Health. Members include Mayo Clinic, Duke University, Harvard Medical School and the University of California, Los Angeles (UCLA). The mission of this organization is to advance the principles and practices of integrative medicine.

In addition, a number of surveys focused on the use of integrative medicine by adults in the United States suggest that more than a third of Americans are already using these practices as part of their health care.

These surveys demonstrate that although the United States has the most advanced medical technology in the world, Americans are turning to integrative treatments — and there are several reasons for this trend. Here are three of the top reasons why more and more people are exploring integrative medicine.

Consumers are more engaged in their health care

One reason integrative medicine is popular is that people in general are taking a greater, more active role in their own health care. People are more aware of health issues and are more open to trying different treatment approaches.

Internet access is also helping to fuel this trend by playing a significant role in improving patient education. Two decades ago, consumers had little access to research or reliable medical information. Today, clinical trials and pharmaceutical developments are more widely available for public knowledge.

For example, people who have arthritis can find a good deal of information about it online. They may find research showing that glucosamine, for example, helps with joint pain and doesn't appear to have a lot of risks associated with it. With this information in hand, they feel empowered to ask their doctors if glucosamine might work with their current treatment plans.

Baby boomers and integrative treatments

A second reason for the wider acceptance of integrative treatments is the influence of the baby boomer generation. This generation is open to a variety of treatments as it explores ways to age well. In addition, baby boomers are often dealing with several medical issues, from weight control to joint pain, high blood pressure and elevated cholesterol. Not everyone wants to start with medication; many prefer to try complementary methods first.

Chronic stress

A third reason for the growth, interest and use of integrative therapies is the degree of chronic stress in the American lifestyle. Workplace stress, long commutes, relationship issues and financial worries are just some of the concerns that make up a long list of stressors.

Although medications can effectively treat short-term stress, they can become just as damag-

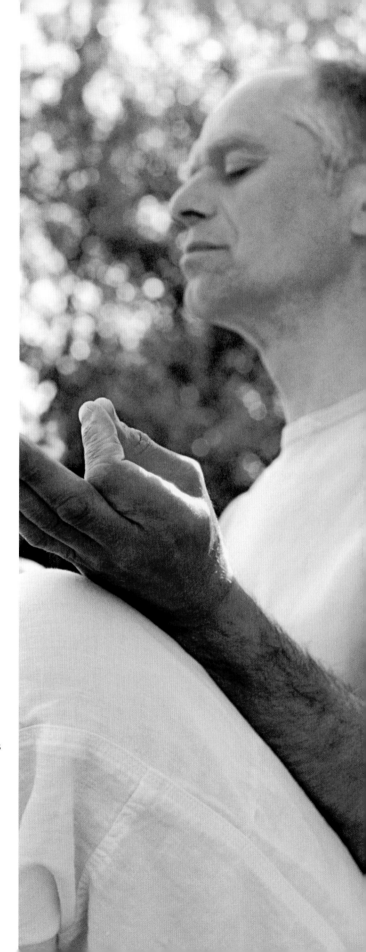

ing — and even as life-threatening — as stress itself is when taken long term. Integrative medicine, on the other hand, offers several effective, evidence-based approaches to dealing with stress that don't involve medication. Many otherwise healthy people are learning to manage the stress in their lives successfully by using complementary methods such as yoga, meditation, massage and guided imagery.

Considering that many healthy people are engaging in integrative practices, it isn't surprising to find out that they're turning to these treatments in times of illness, as well. Here are just a few ways integrative medicine is used to help people cope with medical conditions:

- Meditation can help manage the anxiety and discomfort of medical procedures.
- Massage has been shown to improve recovery rates after heart surgery.
- Gentle tai chi or yoga can assist the transition back to an active life after illness or surgery.

Conventional Western medicine doesn't have cures for everything. Many people who have arthritis, back pain, neck pain, fibromyalgia and anxiety look to integrative treatments to help them manage these often-chronic conditions without the need for medications that may have serious side effects or that may be addictive.

What the research says about integrative medicine

As interest in integrative medicine continues to grow, so does the research in this field. Researchers are studying these approaches in an effort to separate evidence-based, effective therapies from those that don't show effectiveness or may be risky. In the process, this research is helping to identify many genuinely beneficial treatments. In essence, both consumer interest and scientific research have led to further review of these therapies within modern medicine.

As evidence showing the safety and efficacy of many of these therapies grows, physicians are starting to integrate aspects of complementary medicine into conventional medical care. Ultimately, this is what has led to the current term *integrative medicine*.

If you're interested in improving your health, many integrative medicine practices can help. Not only can they speed your recovery from illness or surgery, but they can also help you cope with a

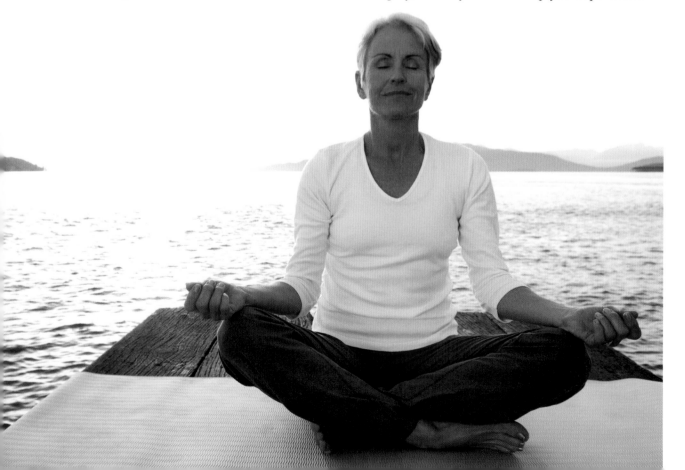

chronic condition. In addition, complementary practices such as meditation and yoga can work to keep you healthy and may actually prevent many diseases.

Throughout this book, you will learn about the integrative practices that show the most promise in terms of safety and effectiveness currently. You'll also learn about the important role you play in maintaining good health with the choices you make each day. In addition, you'll get a firsthand view of how integrative medicine is practiced at Mayo Clinic. Finally, we'll close this book with insights into how you can use what you've learned and start to incorporate it into your daily life.

Integrative vs. alternative: What's the difference?

Alternative medicine is used *in place of* conventional medicine. An example of an alternative therapy is using a special diet to treat cancer in place of undergoing surgery, radiation or chemotherapy that has been recommended by a conventional doctor.

Integrative medicine, on the other hand, *combines* mainstream medical treatments and complementary therapies that have scientific evidence behind safety and efficacy. An example of an integrative therapy is using acupuncture to help lessen nausea after surgery.

Integrative medicine and health

"Integrative medicine and health reaffirms the importance of the relationship between practitioner and patient, focuses on the whole person, is informed by evidence, and makes use of all appropriate therapeutic and lifestyle approaches, healthcare professionals and disciplines to achieve optimal health and healing."

Source:
Academic Consortium for Integrative Medicine & Health, 2017

Expert insight

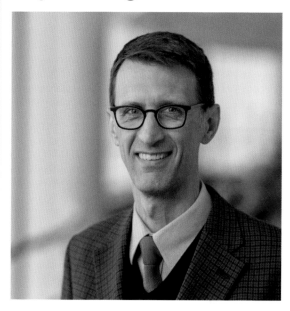

Jon C. Tilburt, M.D.
General Internal Medicine

Dr. Tilburt practices medicine as part of the integrative medicine program at Mayo Clinic in Rochester, Minnesota.

Integrative medicine has gone by several different names over the years, all aiming to describe something that is separate from conventional medicine. But it's much more than that. It's an open-minded, patient-centered pragmatism about whole-person health.

As health care reform continues to be discussed, health organizations are seeing integrative medicine as a way to help prevent chronic disease and promote good health. A report from the National Academy of Medicine suggests that integrative health — in using the best, evidence-based approaches to care — can empower each one of us to build our own wellness and partner with our health care teams to do that effectively.

Integrative medicine at Mayo Clinic

Mayo Clinic Integrative Medicine and Health was developed almost 20 years ago to address interest by patients in products and practices not typically part of conventional medical care. Specially trained doctors and other health professionals work with patients and their doctors to provide information on integrative therapies and to encourage healing and wellness through a variety of channels.

The following treatments promoted through Mayo Clinic Integrative Medicine and Health aren't substitutes for conventional medical care. They're used in concert with standard medical treatment to help alleviate signs and symptoms and conditions and to help promote a sense of well-being.

Massage

Massage is used in a variety of settings at Mayo Clinic. Individuals experiencing pain and other symptoms related to fibromyalgia, migraines, or back or neck problems may receive massage therapy. Massage is also used by patients and staff to reduce stress and anxiety. You may even receive a massage before or after surgery — to help reduce preoperative anxiety and postoperative pain and nausea.

Meditation

At Mayo Clinic, individuals are taught how to meditate and then are given tools to help them perfect the technique on their own.

Acupuncture

At Mayo Clinic, licensed acupuncturists use acupuncture to treat a variety of conditions and symptoms, ranging from back, neck and shoulder pain to fibromyalgia and infertility. A Mayo Clinic study found that a single acupuncture session also can reduce nausea after surgery.

Music therapy

Mayo Clinic has been using music therapy for patients in the hospital for many years. As with other integrative therapies, music therapy is used with conventional medical approaches.

Stress management

Stress Management and Resiliency Training (SMART) is a structured program that has been scientifically proven to reduce symptoms of stress and anxiety and increase well-being, resilience, self-regulation, mindfulness, happiness and positive health behavior.

Participants in the SMART program learn how to train their attention so that it's stronger and it's more focused in the present moment. They learn to guide their thoughts based on higher principles rather than by prejudices. The program has been tested in 20 completed research studies at and outside of Mayo Clinic, with the results showing a decrease in stress and anxiety and an improvement in positive health behaviors. Learn about one of these studies below.

Case study: How SMART works

Mayo Clinic tested the SMART program on newly licensed nurses going through orientation, one of the most stressful times during a registered nurse's career. Researchers asked half of the nurses to take a 90-minute class that taught them basic mind-body skills and how to interpret things in a positive way.

The nurses in this group learned about stress and resilience in the mind and the body. They also learned about mind-body techniques they could use to manage stress, including:
- Training their attention
- Focusing on higher meaning

- Practicing gratitude, compassion, acceptance and forgiveness

The second group of nurses attended a lecture about the nursing orientation program. As part of this lecture, these nurses learned about topics related to stress, including work-life connectedness.

Researchers followed all of the nurses in both groups for a year and found that the nurses who were trained in the SMART approach and practiced its mind-body techniques were happier with their jobs and were less stressed.

Top integrative treatments

What are some of the most promising practices in integrative medicine? Here's a list of 10 treatments that you might consider for your own health and wellness. All of them are used at Mayo Clinic, and you'll learn about each of them in this book.

- **Acupuncture** is a Chinese practice that involves inserting very thin needles at strategic points on the body. Learn about acupuncture starting on page 94.
- **Guided imagery** involves bringing to mind a specific image or a series of memories to produce certain responses in the body. Learn about guided imagery starting on page 64.
- **Hypnotherapy** involves a trancelike state where the mind is more open to suggestion. Learn about hypnotherapy starting on page 69.
- **Massage** uses pressure to manipulate the soft tissues of the body. There are many different kinds of massage, and some have specific health goals in mind. Learn about massage therapy starting on page 82.
- **Meditation** involves clearing and calming the mind by focusing on your breathing or a word, phrase or sound. Learn about meditation starting on page 56.
- **Music therapy** can influence both your mental and physical health. Learn about music therapy starting on page 50.
- **Spinal manipulation,** which is also called spinal adjustment, is practiced by chiropractors and physical therapists. Learn about spinal manipulation starting on page 76.
- **Spirituality** has many definitions, but its focus is on an individual's connection to others and to the search for meaning in life. Learn about spirituality starting on page 72.
- **Tai chi** is a graceful exercise in which you move from pose to pose. You'll see tai chi mentioned throughout this book, as well as highlighted on page 29.
- **Yoga** involves a series of postures that often include a focus on breathing. Yoga is commonly practiced to relieve stress, as well as treat heart disease and depression. You'll see yoga mentioned throughout this book and highlighted on page 29.

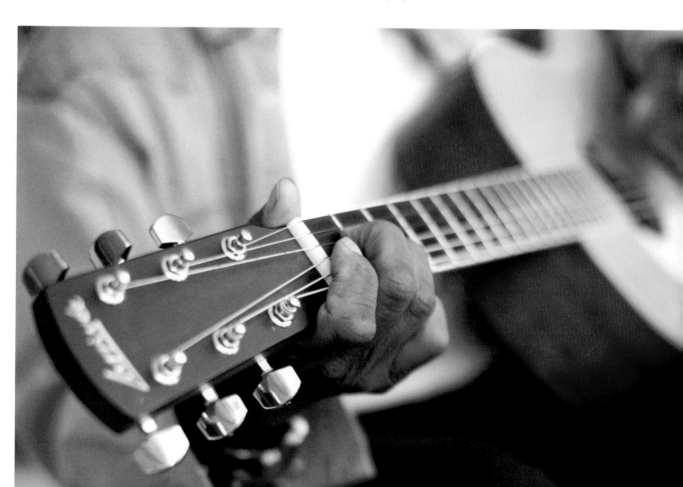

Build your wellness foundation first

Before you begin to learn about integrative approaches, take a moment to think about your personal wellness. No approach — conventional or integrative — can help you reach your health goals if you don't take steps to build your foundation of wellness first.

The basic components of a healthy life — nutrition, exercise, stress management and a strong support network — provide your wellness foundation. Without these basics, no medical intervention will work as well. No integrative approach can take the place of these basic tenets of personal wellness. You'll learn more about the steps you can take to build a solid wellness foundation starting on page 18.

Building your wellness foundation is the first step you can take to help prevent health issues in the first place. This is one place where integrative medicine can help.

For example, integrative therapies and techniques can help you reduce stress, eat well, and

improve your balance and muscle tone. These are all steps you can take to improve your health and prevent illness.

If, after reading the next section in this book, you feel as though you have a solid wellness foundation in place but still have a persisting symptom or problem, integrative medicine may be appropriate. That's when targeted, evidence-based integrative therapies may be worth looking into and discussing with your health care team.

As you embark on your journey toward better health, start with the basics. For example, try eating less fast food and more fruits and vegetables. Relax with a warm bath or a few minutes of quiet reflection. Go for a daily walk around the neighborhood. And get together with friends you enjoy and can really talk to. Every step you take to improve your personal wellness is a step toward living a longer and more enjoyable life.

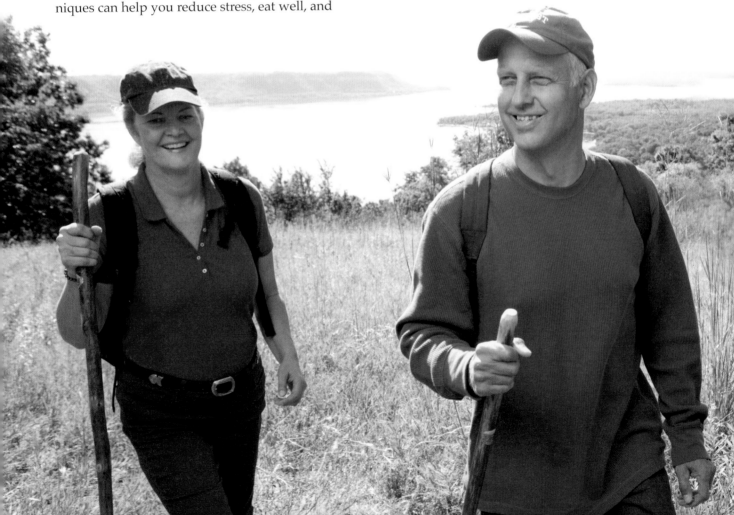

How to use this resource

Doctors and other staff in Integrative Medicine and Health at Mayo Clinic developed this publication to provide you straightforward information about various therapies being used and what's known about them.

With each treatment included in this book, you will learn about the latest research, the safety and effectiveness of the product or practice, and any potential risks.

You will also continue to read about lifestyle habits that can help you build a solid wellness foundation and how they can help ensure that you get the most out of the efforts you're making to improve your health.

The *Mayo Clinic Guide to Integrative Medicine* is a personal health guide that can help you achieve great health and fully enjoy life.

About the lights

A special feature of this part of the book — which you'll find in upcoming pages — is our stoplight. Its purpose is to give you an at-a-glance overview as to how you should proceed with the therapy being discussed.

A shining red light means not to use the treatment or to use it very carefully and only under a doctor's close supervision. A therapy is given a red light when studies have found it to be unsafe or have found its risks far outweigh any benefits it may provide.

A shining yellow light means to use the therapy with caution. A treatment is given a yellow light when studies show it may be of benefit but that it also carries some risks. Therapies that have not been fully studied to determine their safety and effectiveness are also given a yellow light. In addition, a treatment may be given a yellow light if it's considered safe, but studies haven't found it to provide any benefit.

A shining green light means the therapy is generally safe for most people to use, and studies show it to be effective. (If you have a specific health condition, a therapy given a green light may not be appropriate for you.) Even when a green light is present, it's still important that you discuss the treatment with your doctor and use it appropriately.

Making wellness the focus of care

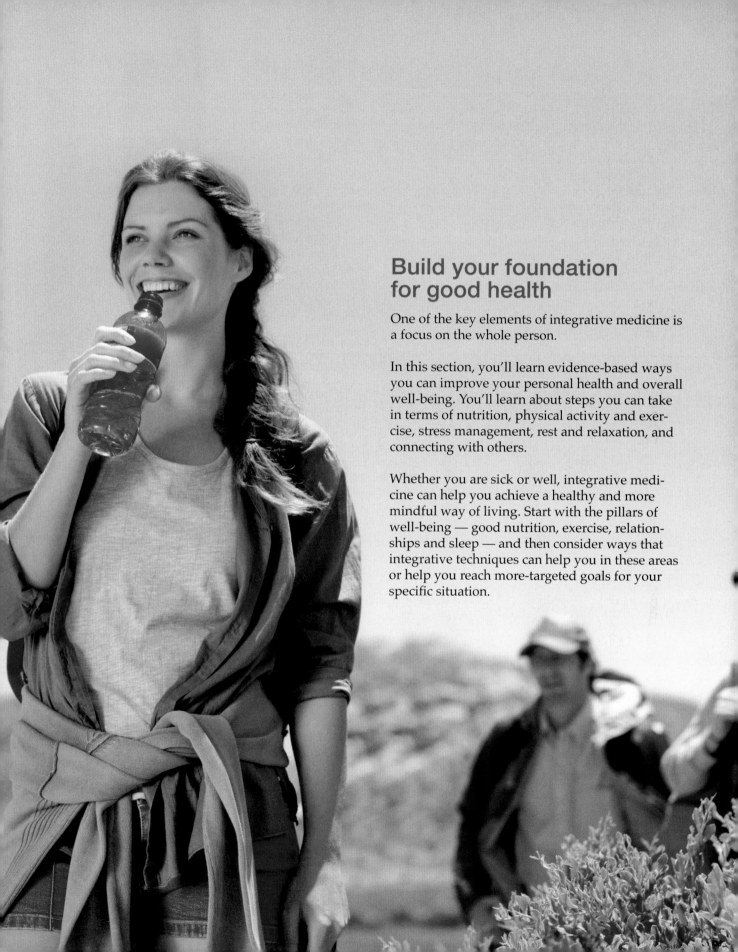

Build your foundation for good health

One of the key elements of integrative medicine is a focus on the whole person.

In this section, you'll learn evidence-based ways you can improve your personal health and overall well-being. You'll learn about steps you can take in terms of nutrition, physical activity and exercise, stress management, rest and relaxation, and connecting with others.

Whether you are sick or well, integrative medicine can help you achieve a healthy and more mindful way of living. Start with the pillars of well-being — good nutrition, exercise, relationships and sleep — and then consider ways that integrative techniques can help you in these areas or help you reach more-targeted goals for your specific situation.

What are your biggest health threats?

Why is it important to know what threatens your health? It's not to scare you, but rather to help guide you in the choices you make regarding your health and safety.

What should you work hardest to avoid? Check out the biggest risks to your health and well-being in the table below and on the next page. You may be surprised to see how many lifestyle choices you can make to boost your odds of living a longer and healthier life — all by taking simple steps every day to reduce your risk of these leading causes of death.

This list also offers one more important opportunity: a chance to see how integrative medicine can help improve your odds of living a longer, more enjoyable life.

For example, you'll notice that managing stress is one lifestyle choice you can make to help reduce your risk of almost all of these leading causes of death. Managing your stress is one choice you can make now that can help reduce your risk of developing several different diseases and conditions in the future.

Beginning in this section and throughout this book, you'll learn how integrative medicine can help you make healthy lifestyle choices, improve your overall wellness and improve your odds of living a long and enjoyable life.

Top 10 leading causes of death in the United States

Cause of death	Lifestyle choices that can help reduce your risk
1. Heart disease	• Don't smoke or use tobacco. • Exercise for about 30 minutes a day, most days of the week. • Follow a diet that's rich in fruits, vegetables and whole grains. • Maintain a healthy weight. • Get enough good-quality sleep. • Manage stress. • Get regular health screenings for blood pressure and cholesterol levels, and blood sugar levels.
2. Cancer	• Don't smoke or use tobacco. • Eat a healthy diet that includes plenty of fruits and vegetables and limits processed meats and high-calorie foods, including refined sugars and fat from animal sources. Drink alcohol in moderation, if at all. • Maintain a healthy weight. • Get regular physical activity. • Protect yourself from the sun. • Get immunized against certain viral infections, such as hepatitis B and human papillomavirus (HPV).
3. Chronic lower respiratory disease	• Don't smoke, and avoid exposure to secondhand tobacco smoke. • Avoid exposure to home and workplace air pollutants. • Wash your hands regularly with soap and water to prevent contracting a respiratory infection. • If you're having breathing problems, ask your doctor if testing to detect a respiratory disease is right for you. • Eat a healthy diet. Some research shows that healthy-eating strategies for preventing other health conditions, including heart disease, diabetes and cancer, can help prevent chronic respiratory disease as well.

4. Accidents (unintentional injuries)	• Wear safety gear, such as a life jacket or the right helmet for your activity. • Look for and remove tripping hazards around your house. • Learn how to swim. • Take medication only as directed and store it out of reach of children. • Place children in the proper booster or car seat. • Wear your seat belt. • Walk on a sidewalk, when possible.
5. Stroke	• Prevent or manage high blood pressure (hypertension). • Reduce the amount of cholesterol and saturated fat in your diet. • Don't smoke or use tobacco; if you do, quit. • Prevent or manage diabetes. • Maintain a healthy weight. • Eat a diet rich in fruits and vegetables. • Drink alcohol in moderation, if at all. • Get treated for obstructive sleep apnea if you have it. • Avoid illicit drugs.
6. Alzheimer's disease	Although there's currently no proven way to prevent Alzheimer's disease, research suggests that you may be able to lower your risk by reducing your risk of heart disease (see heart disease prevention strategies on previous page).
7. Diabetes	• Eat healthy foods – especially fruits, vegetables and whole grains, as well as foods that are lower in fat and calories and higher in fiber. • Aim for at least 30 minutes of moderate physical activity a day. • Reach and maintain a healthy weight.
8. Flu (influenza) and pneumonia	To reduce the risk of the flu: • Get an annual flu vaccination. • Wash your hands regularly. • Cover your mouth and nose when you sneeze and cough. • Avoid crowds during peak flu season. To reduce your risk of pneumonia: • Ask your doctor if a pneumonia vaccination makes sense for you. • Wash your hands regularly. • Don't smoke.
9. Kidney disease	• Take over-the-counter medications only as directed. • Maintain a healthy weight. • Don't smoke. • Manage medical conditions that increase your risk of kidney disease.
10. Suicide	• **Get the treatment you need.** You may feel embarrassed to seek treatment for mental health problems, but getting the right treatment for depression, substance misuse or another underlying problem will make you feel better about life — and help keep you safe. • **Establish your support network.** It may be hard to talk about suicidal feelings, and your friends and family may not fully understand why you feel the way you do. Reach out anyway, and make sure the people who care about you are there when you need them. Consider getting help from your place of worship, support groups or other community resources. Feeling connected and supported can help reduce suicide risk. • **Remember, suicidal feelings are temporary.** If you feel hopeless or that life's not worth living anymore, remember that treatment can help you regain your perspective — and life will get better. Take one step at a time and don't act impulsively.

Nutrition

Over the years, many popular diets have come and gone, but a handful of diets you may be familiar with have been proved to be effective in improving health. Here's a little background on several popular diets.

Mediterranean diet and DASH diet

You're likely familiar with the Mediterranean diet and the Dietary Approaches to Stop Hypertension (DASH) diet. Both of these diets:

- Help prevent high cholesterol, high blood pressure and heart disease
- Emphasize whole grains, fruits and vegetables, nuts, olive oil, fish and poultry
- Offer plenty of variety in an effort to help you improve your lifelong eating habits
- Do not ban sweets, red meat or alcohol, but do limit them to small amounts
- Can help you reach a healthy weight as a side benefit, though neither focuses on weight loss

Although these two diets share many similarities, the DASH diet places more emphasis on lowering sodium intake and on portion control.

What the research says

Both the Mediterranean and DASH diets have been proved in study after study to reduce the risk of heart disease, as well as diabetes and some types of cancer. If strictly followed, they may even help prevent or slow the progression of Alzheimer's disease. The Mediterranean and DASH diets have been scientifically proved to be the best diets to achieve long-term health and wellness. Studies have even shown that these diets reduce the risk of stroke, heart disease and dementia.

MIND diet

In 2015, Rush University Medical Center released a study on the Mediterranean-DASH Intervention for Neurodegenerative Delay (MIND diet). The MIND diet is based on the Mediterranean and DASH diets, but it focuses specifically on brain health.

The MIND diet recommends 10 brain-healthy foods and restricts five foods that aren't as healthy.

The 10 brain-healthy foods are:
- Green leafy vegetables (a salad every day)
- Other vegetables (in addition to eating a salad every day)
- Nuts (every other day or so)
- Berries (at least twice a week; blueberries especially, but also strawberries)
- Beans (every other day or so)
- Whole grains (at least three servings a day)
- Fish (at least once a week)
- Poultry (at least twice a week)
- Olive oil
- Wine (one 5-ounce glass a day)

The five unhealthy foods are:
- Red meats (less than a serving a week)
- Butter and stick margarine (less than a tablespoon a day)
- Cheese (less than a serving a week)
- Pastries and sweets (less than a serving a week)
- Fried or fast food (less than a serving a week for each)

What the research says

Researchers who studied more than 900 people between the ages of 58 and 98 for four and a half years found that those who closely followed the MIND diet reduced their incidence of Alzheimer's disease by 50 percent. Those who moderately followed the diet reduced their risk by 35 percent.

The Mayo Clinic Diet

Mayo Clinic has developed a diet designed to help those who follow it lose weight and achieve the health benefits that a healthy weight offers, called the Mayo Clinic Diet.

Developed by Mayo Clinic health experts and first published in a book of the same name in 2010, the Mayo Clinic Diet is a weight-loss and lifestyle program designed to help people lose weight by adopting lifestyle habits that they can maintain long term. Choosing healthy foods and developing healthy lifestyle habits, including regular physical activity, are part of this diet.

The idea behind the Mayo Clinic Diet is that successful, long-term weight control requires a focus on overall health, not just what you eat. It also emphasizes that the best way to manage weight long-term requires changing your lifestyle and adopting new health habits. The Mayo Clinic Diet can be tailored to your own individual needs and situations.

Which diet is right for you?

No one dietary approach is best for every person. As you consider what changes you want to make in your eating habits, consider which parts of these diets may help you improve your health and wellness in a way that fits your personal situation best.

For example, try taping a list of the 15 healthy and unhealthy foods from the MIND diet to your refrigerator door. Maybe posting the Mayo Clinic Healthy Weight Pyramid from the Mayo Clinic Diet can help you keep track of what and how much you're eating. Or perhaps trying some new recipes from the Mediterranean diet is just the kick-start you need. Remember: Small changes over time can make a difference.

How you eat

What's on your plate is one important aspect of good nutrition. But *how* you eat is another key to healthy eating. As you think about how you eat, ask yourself these questions:
- Do you eat while doing something else, such as watching television, reading a book, or using a computer or other electronic device?

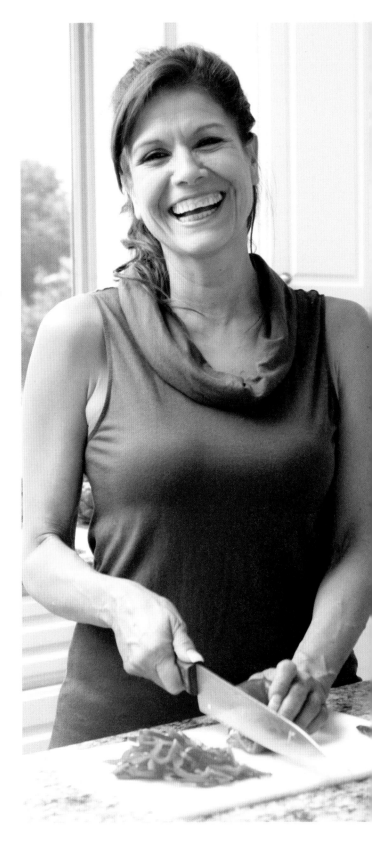

- Do you eat while you're at your desk in the office or in the car on the way to work?
- How much attention do you pay to what you're eating?
- At what pace do you tend to eat? Do you eat slowly, or do you eat quickly?

Depending on how you answered these questions, practicing mindfulness at your next meal may be another way that you can improve your eating habits.

Mindfulness means different things to different people, but in a traditional sense, it means being present in the moment. Eating mindfully means taking time to eat and becoming fully aware of the tastes and the textures of the food in your mouth. By doing this, you slow down, giving your body a chance to tell you when you're full. Other ways to try mindfulness include putting your fork down or taking sips of water between each bite.

Eat for your health

What you eat has a direct effect on how you feel and how your body functions. A healthy diet — one that emphasizes vegetables, fruits and whole grains — may lower your risk of developing many diseases. The goal is to eat foods that not only taste good, but are good for you.

Vegetables and fruits

Every day, researchers learn more and more about how vegetables and fruits supply the body with a variety of substances to ward off illness.

People who typically eat generous helpings of vegetables and fruits are at lower risk of developing many leading causes of death, including:
- Heart disease
- High blood pressure
- Cancer
- Diabetes

Carbohydrates

When it comes to carbohydrates, the key word to remember is *whole*, as in *whole grains*. The less

refined a carbohydrate food is, the better it is for your health. Whole grains abound with vitamins, minerals and other important nutrients.

Choose whole-grain breads, pastas and cereals whenever you can, and select brown rice instead of white rice.

Protein and dairy

Despite what you may have learned early on in life, it's not necessary to eat meat every day. Although meat is rich in protein, many cuts of meat are high in saturated fat and cholesterol. When you do eat meat, try to eat only lean cuts.

A variety of other foods furnish protein, too, including:
- Low-fat dairy products
- Seafood
- Legumes (dried beans, lentils and peas)

Try to substitute these foods for meat on a regular basis. These foods provide other benefits, as well. For example, low-fat dairy products are rich in calcium and vitamin D, and seafood supplies omega-3 fatty acids, which help protect against heart disease.

Fats

Not all fats are bad for you. Nuts, for instance, contain vitamin E, which helps keep your heart and arteries free from harmful deposits. And research shows that people who replace much of the animal fat in their meals with liquid vegetable oils, such as olive or canola oil, can reduce their blood cholesterol level.

While nuts and products such as vegetable oil may be beneficial to your health, they are high in calories, so it's best to use them in moderation.

Sweets

You don't have to give up sweets entirely to eat well, but be smart about your selections and portion sizes. Small portions of chocolate — especially dark chocolate — contain antioxidants that may even provide some health benefits.

Getting into a healthy groove

With everything that you have to do each day, making sure that you and your family eat healthy meals may seem difficult and time-consuming.

When it comes to cooking, many people claim that they don't have the time. That's because healthy eating is often associated with complicated recipes, time-laden meal preparation and hours spent at the grocery store. However, you can prepare a healthy meal as quickly as you can an unhealthy one. Here are several ways you can eat well without a lot of fuss and hassle.

Plan by the week

It can be more efficient to plan meals for an entire week, especially if you shop for groceries on a weekly basis. Planning your meals each week will help ensure that you have all of the right ingredients on hand when it's time to prepare breakfast, lunch or dinner.

Look for shortcuts

Another way to help simplify meal preparation and save time is to purchase pre-cut vegetables and fruits, precooked meats, and packaged salads. Frozen or canned vegetables also may come in handy for some dishes. Rinse the canned vegetables to help remove the sodium used in processing.

Shop from a list

Following a list helps keep you from impulse buying. Avoid shopping when you're hungry — you may be tempted to grab anything that looks vaguely appetizing.

Read nutrition labels

When shopping, compare the nutrition labels of similar items to see if one is healthier than the others. You may find that one has less fat, fewer calories or more fiber.

Adapt to the seasons

Whenever you can, look for recently harvested produce. Here are several examples:
- Spring: asparagus, peas, cherries
- Midsummer: peaches, sweet corn, tomatoes
- Fall: apples, pears, squash

In the spring, summer and early fall months, look for farmers markets near you. Farmers markets offer local produce, which tends to be the freshest around.

Be adventurous

Discovering new foods and flavors is part of the joy of cooking and eating, so don't be afraid to explore unfamiliar cuisines. Keep in mind that the broadest range of health benefits comes from meals that feature a wide variety of foods.

Be flexible

Remember that every food you eat doesn't have to be an excellent source of nutrients. Nor is it out of the question to eat high-fat, high-calorie foods on occasion. The main thing is that you choose foods that promote good health more often than you choose those that don't.

Exercise

Starting a fitness program may be one of the best things you can do for your health. Starting a fitness program is an important decision, but it doesn't have to be an overwhelming one. By planning carefully and pacing yourself, you can make fitness a healthy habit that lasts a lifetime.

A move toward wellness

Although it's not surprising that physical activity and structured exercise offer many health benefits, it bears repeating simply because researchers have found that moving more affects all aspects of your health — mind, body and spirit.

The following is a sampling of what researchers have learned about the benefits of exercise and physical activity.

Aerobic exercise and cognitive health

Several studies have shown that aerobic exercise, such as walking, bicycling, swimming and dancing, reduce age-related brain shrinkage while improving memory and other cognitive functions.

For example, a study of 120 older adults found that aerobic exercise increases the size of the brain that's involved in spatial memory, improving how well this area of the brain functions.

Other studies show that aerobic exercise increases the size of the hippocampus, a part of the brain associated with memory, and improves memory in people with multiple sclerosis.

And finally, researchers who studied the effect of exercise on older men with coronary artery disease found a link between exercise and increased density of gray matter in the brain.

Heart and lung strength

Physical activity offers specific benefits in terms of how your heart and lungs operate. For example, it:

- Reduces the buildup of harmful deposits in your arteries by increasing the concentration of high-density lipoprotein (HDL or "good") cholesterol in your blood.
- Strengthens your heart so that it can pump blood more efficiently. That, in turn, reduces the risk of developing high blood pressure.

Disease prevention

Exercise helps prevent several diseases and conditions. It keeps bones and muscles strong by maintaining bone density, which plays several roles in preventing osteoporosis. It also helps you reach and maintain a healthy weight, which improves diseases and conditions associated with being overweight, such as diabetes. Exercise also appears to reduce your risk of certain cancers — colon, prostate, breast, uterine lining cancers and maybe others.

A better night's sleep

In part by increasing serotonin, moderate exercise at least three hours before bedtime can help you relax and sleep better at night. In turn, a good night's sleep helps maintain your physical and mental health.

Immune system and illness

Although larger studies are needed to confirm these findings, some research shows that moderate aerobic exercise may help prevent the common cold.

Researchers who have found that exercise does help suggest that it has a positive effect on the cells that impact the immune system.

Emotional health

Exercise can accomplish many of the same things that medications are designed to do. For example, from a psychological standpoint, exercise raises endorphins, which boosts energy.

Physical activity also offers a sense of accomplishment. For example, if at first you could walk only 10 minutes at a time, but now you can walk for 15 minutes, you may feel more motivated to keep pushing forward.

A connection to others

Team fitness activities and sports naturally involve other people, so in these cases, exercise enhances connections with other people.

But team-based sports and activities aren't the only ways that physical activity brings people together. For example, one researcher studied a large cross-country ski race in Minnesota. The researcher found that even in this solo sport, athletes developed a strong community, sharing exercise tips and recipes.

A spiritual experience

Some runners say that running in the woods helps them become more mindful and aware. Other people find a spiritual component when they're enjoying a day on a lake in a kayak or a canoe.

Before you start

If you haven't exercised in a while or are starting a new exercise routine and have health issues or concerns, talk to your doctor. Find a list of exercise cautions on page 30.

Setting fitness goals

No matter how fit you are, setting goals can help keep you motivated and enjoying physical activity. If you're starting a new exercise program, think first about how fit you are and then plan your physical activity — how much you will do and how often you will do it — based on your fitness level right now, as well as your goals. Your health care team can help you set goals that are reasonable for your situation.

As a first step, test how physically fit you are with the short assessment on the next page.

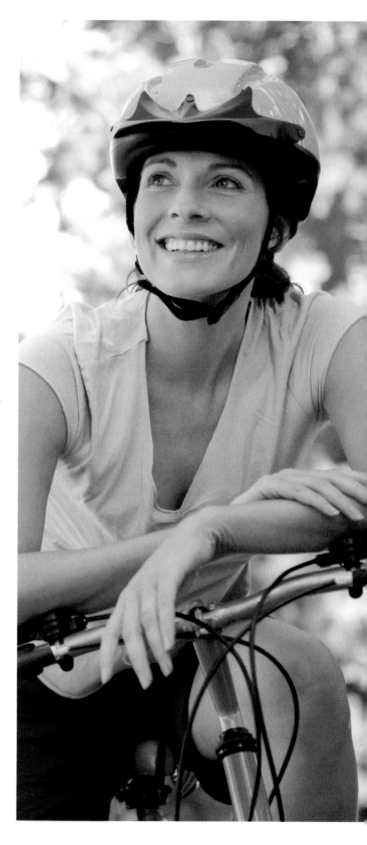

Assess your physical fitness

Before starting a physical activity program, take this short assessment. Write down your answers to the following and gauge your results by searching on "fitness test" on *www.MayoClinic.org*.

1. Your pulse rate before and after walking 1 mile
2. How long it takes you to walk 1 mile
3. How many pushups you can do at a time
4. How far you can reach forward while seated on the floor with your legs in front of you
5. Your waist circumference as measured around your bare abdomen just above your hipbones
6. Your body mass index (Visit *www.MayoClinic. org* and search on "BMI" to find a calculator.)

Design your fitness program

After you've tested how physically fit you are right now, take time to consider what physical activity routine you will enjoy — and what will help you reach your wellness goals.

Start designing your personal fitness program by asking yourself the following questions.

What are my fitness goals?

Do you want to lose weight? Or, do you have another motivation, such as preparing for a marathon? Having clear goals — and writing them down — can help you gauge your progress.

What amount of exercise should I work toward?

Each week, most adults should aim for at least 150 minutes of moderate-intensity aerobic activity, 75 minutes of vigorous aerobic activity, or a combination of the two. It's also important to aim for two or more days of strength training a week.

At the same time, keep in mind that many people start exercising too long or too intensely — and give up when their muscles and joints become sore or injured. Plan time between sessions for your body to rest and recover.

What pace should I aim for?

If you are just beginning to exercise or haven't exercised in a while, start cautiously and progress slowly. If you have an injury or a medical condition, talk to your doctor or a physical therapist for help designing a fitness program that gradually improves your range of motion, strength and endurance.

Give yourself time to warm up and cool down with easy walking or gentle stretching. Then speed up to a pace you can continue for five to 10 minutes without getting overly tired. As your stamina improves, gradually increase the amount of time you exercise. Work your way up to 30 to 60 minutes of exercise most days of the week.

Finally, remember to listen to your body. If you're not feeling well, give yourself permission to take a day or two off. And if you feel pain, shortness of breath, dizziness or nausea during exercise, take a break. You may be pushing yourself too hard.

How can I build activity into my daily routine?

Schedule time to exercise as you would any other appointment. Plan to watch your favorite show while walking on a treadmill, or read while riding a stationary bike. Also, keep in mind that you don't have to do all your exercise at one time. Shorter but more-frequent sessions have aerobic benefits, too.

How can I keep my exercise routine interesting?

A little creativity can go a long way. Consider a workout routine that includes various activities, such as walking, bicycling or rowing. But don't stop there. Take a weekend hike with your family or spend an evening ballroom dancing.

Or involve several different activities through cross-training. Cross-training also reduces your chances of injuring or overusing one specific muscle or joint. Plan to alternate among activities that emphasize different parts of your body, such as walking, swimming and strength training.

Integrative physical activity techniques

Once you have a good idea of how fit you are and what steps you want to take toward getting more physically active, the next step is to choose activities that make the most sense for you.

If you are struggling to make a commitment to getting regular exercise, taking a less traditional approach may help. Integrative forms of physical activity may offer the boost you need to get regular physical activity — and even enjoy it.

These exercises may not satisfy all of your aerobic activity needs, but they can help you enjoy a variety of different types of physical activity.

Yoga

Yoga can help you improve your balance, flexibility, range of motion and strength. As with other types of physical activity, yoga can help reduce your risk of chronic diseases, such as heart disease and high blood pressure. It can also help you manage chronic conditions, such as depression, pain, anxiety and insomnia.

Researchers also have found that people who participate in yoga feel more confident about their ability to exercise, which can lead to an increase in sticking with a physical activity program. In one study of overweight adults who were getting little or no physical activity, researchers found that yoga was a "stepping stone" toward regular exercise, helping people stick to a regular physical activity program.

Tai chi

Tai chi is a self-paced, mind-body intervention. It incorporates gentle stretching, deep breathing and relaxation exercises with physical activity that's low or moderate in intensity. Because it's low impact, tai chi is generally safe for all ages and fitness levels.

Tai chi has been shown to help improve aerobic exercise capacity in older adults who get little to no regular physical activity. Research also shows that participating in tai chi can help people feel more capable of getting regular physical activity. Tai chi has also been shown to improve quality of life and mood in adults with heart failure.

Pilates

Pilates can help you build strength in your core muscles, which helps lead to better posture, core strength, stability, balance and flexibility. It involves low-impact flexibility, strength training and endurance movements.

As with tai chi and yoga, researchers have found that Pilates is another type of physical activity that can help improve your self-confidence in committing to getting regular physical activity.

Qi gong

Qi gong involves slow and rhythmic movements designed to help teach balance and increase flexibility. It can improve bone health, how well the heart and lungs work, and balance, as well as quality of life and even chronic pain.

In a review of the health benefits of qi gong and tai chi, researchers found that qi gong enhanced not only people's belief in being able to exercise regularly, but also helped them feel better able to handle stress and new experiences.

What does being fit mean to you?

Being fit means different things to different people. Feeling fit may mean doing all the activities you want to without discomfort. Or it may mean that your heart rate slows to a healthy level, your blood pressure is well-controlled, and your blood sugar is at a healthy level. These are just a few of the many ways that you can gauge what being fit means to you.

In the end, keep in mind that everyone is built differently and has different motivations when it comes to physical fitness. Consider finding a daily activity you like to do and work from there. That in itself is one step toward wellness.

Exercise cautions

Talk to your doctor before you start an exercise program if you:
- Have heart disease
- Have asthma or lung disease
- Have type 1 or type 2 diabetes
- Have kidney disease
- Have arthritis
- Are being treated for cancer, or you have recently completed cancer treatment

Check with your doctor if you have any of these signs or symptoms, which may suggest that you have heart, lung or other serious disease:
- Pain or discomfort in your chest, neck, jaw or arms during physical activity
- Dizziness, lightheadedness or fainting with exercise or exertion
- Shortness of breath with mild exertion, at rest, or when lying down or going to bed
- Ankle swelling, especially at night
- A rapid or pronounced heartbeat
- A heart murmur that your doctor has previously diagnosed
- Lower leg pain when you walk, which goes away with rest

The American College of Sports Medicine recommends that you see your doctor before engaging in vigorous exercise if two or more of the following apply:
- You're older than 35.
- You have a family history of heart disease before age 60.
- You smoke or you quit smoking in the past six months.
- You don't normally exercise for at least 30 minutes, most days of the week.
- You're significantly overweight.
- You have high blood pressure or high cholesterol.
- You have type 1 or type 2 diabetes, or you have impaired glucose tolerance (also known as prediabetes).

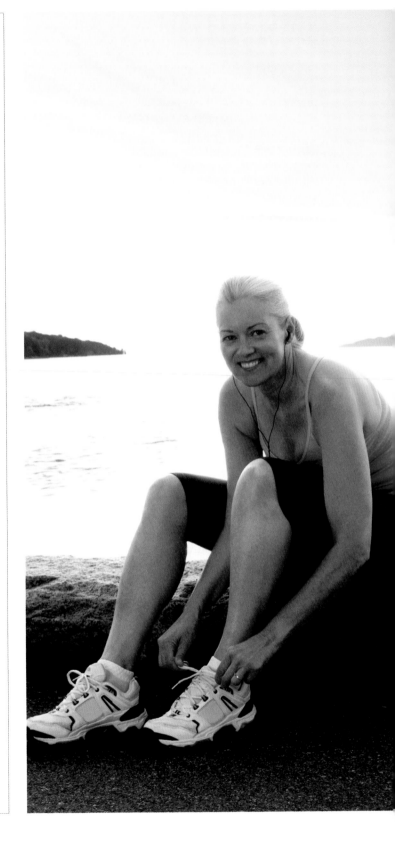

Stress

You catch yourself clenching your fists or your jaw. Your tense muscles are causing your neck or shoulders to hurt. Your stomach is upset. You have a headache. You have trouble sleeping. You eat when you're not hungry. You skip exercise. Your temper is short, even with the people you love the most.

These are just some examples of common — but unhealthy — reactions to stress. Do any of these scenarios sound like you?

How stress affects your body

Your body is hard-wired to respond to stress in ways that don't fit the types of stress faced by most people today. This reaction is known as the fight-or-flight response, and it happens naturally without your having to think about it. Your body automatically pumps up your heart rate, increases blood flow to the muscles you need, and shuts off blood flow to less vital body functions.

Here's a step-by-step look at what happens in your body when it's faced with stress:

- Your adrenal glands, which sit on top of your kidneys, release a surge of hormones, including adrenaline and cortisol, your body's main stress hormone.
- Adrenaline increases your heart rate, raises your blood pressure and boosts the amount of energy available for your body to use.
- Cortisol increases the sugars in your bloodstream, enhances your brain's use of it and makes sure that your body has enough tissue-repairing substances available.
- Cortisol also curbs the bodily functions that you don't need in a fight-or-flight situation. Your immune system, digestive system, reproductive system and growth processes are all affected.

Stress also affects your heart in another way: It affects your *heart rate variability*. Put simply, two parts of your autonomic nervous system keep the balance of your heart rate healthy. Without this balance, these two parts of your autonomic nervous system kick into overdrive. This, in turn, increases your risk of heart disease — and, by extension, many other types of disease. (See "What is heart rate variability?" on page 33 to learn more.)

Your body's natural response to stress can be helpful and, at times, lifesaving. But it isn't always necessary these days, because most of the stress in today's world isn't life-threatening. However, your body doesn't know this — so when you get in an argument, for example, your body's instinct is to protect you. It sends a boost of adrenaline through your body, and your heart rate increases.

This reaction isn't going to help you cope with most of the stressors you face today, but this is your body's way of protecting you against threats — threats that are rare today.

In most cases, once your stress — what your body thinks is a threat — has passed, everything in your body returns to normal. But some people always feel stressed, which means that this fight-or-flight response is always turned on.

If your fight-or-flight response is always turned on, over time too much exposure to cortisol and other stress hormones can increase your risk of:

- Anxiety
- Depression
- Digestive problems
- Headaches
- Heart disease
- Sleep problems
- Weight gain
- Memory and concentration impairment

Steps toward less stress

Because such a large part of today's modern lifestyle revolves around stress, it's crucial to find healthy ways to manage it.

To start, take an honest look at how you naturally react to stress. Do you eat unhealthy foods? Lash out at others in anger? Get headaches or stomachaches? Reactions like these — as well as those at the beginning of this section — will help you see opportunities where you can improve how you respond to stress.

From there, use these self-management strategies to improve how you manage stress.

- **Practice self-care.** Make healthy food choices and get regular exercise and enough good-quality sleep.
- **Scale back when you can.** Take a close look at your daily, weekly and monthly schedule and find meetings, activities, dinners or chores that you can cut back on or delegate to someone else.
- **Try relaxation techniques.** Yoga, deep breathing and meditation are all examples. It doesn't matter which relaxation technique you choose. What matters is refocusing your attention to something calming and increasing awareness of your body.
- **Take time for hobbies,** such as reading a book or listening to music — things that you don't get competitive or more stressed out about. When you engage in something enjoyable, it can soothe and calm your mind.
- **Connect with others.** Keep in touch with supportive, caring people in your social circle.
- **Nurture your spirituality.** Cultivating your spirituality can help you uncover what's most meaningful in your life, realize that you aren't responsible for everything in life, feel a sense of connection to something larger than yourself, and even expand your social network.
- **Keep your sense of humor.** Laughter really is good medicine — it can help you when you're facing stress, but it also offers long-term benefits.
- **Volunteer in your community.** When you help others by devoting time to a cause you care about, you may find that you're helping yourself, too.
- **Get professional help when needed.** If your stress management efforts aren't helpful enough, see your doctor.

Although stress usually doesn't get better on its own, you can actively take steps to manage stress in a way that allows you to live your life without stress controlling it.

Beyond the basics

In upcoming pages, you'll read about a number of techniques that can help you relax and reduce stress.

The best thing about mind and body therapies to relieve stress is that they're safe and often effective.

If you're interested in learning about integrative therapies that can help you manage stress, here's a list of options you'll find in this book:

- Biofeedback (see page 66)
- Guided imagery (see page 64)
- Massage (see page 82)
- Meditation (see page 56)
- Progressive muscle relaxation (see page 44)
- Music therapy (see page 50)
- Relaxed breathing (see page 46)

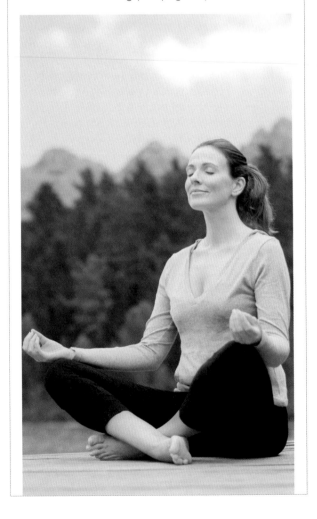

What is heart rate variability?

How much do you know about heart rate variability? Test your knowledge — and learn how it affects your health and how you can improve it.

True or false? The heart plays a complex role in your health.
Answer: True.
Keeping your heart healthy is important for your overall health for a number of reasons, but the role your heart plays in your overall health may be even more complex than once thought. Your heart is a pump, it generates rhythm, it's a sensory organ, and it plays a key role in the communication that takes place throughout your body. Your heart may even play a role in how you interpret your experience of the world around you.

True or false? A healthy heart always beats at a steady rate.
Answer: False.
A healthy heart doesn't always beat at as steady a rate as you may think. Your heart rate is a much more complicated process that's affected by your breathing as well as your environment.

Your heart rate varies from beat to beat. If you see it charted out, you'll notice patterns in your heartbeat. These patterns can be regular or irregular, and the beat-to-beat changes you see in these patterns are known as heart rate variability.

True or false? Heart rate variability can affect your health.
Answer: True.
Let's start with the basics: Put simply, heart rate variability represents the slight variations in the timing of each heartbeat. These variations are caused by an ongoing balancing act that takes place behind the scenes in how your heart beats. This balancing act takes place between the two branches of your autonomic nervous system: your sympathetic and parasympathetic nervous systems.

When you face a threat, the sympathetic nervous system helps your body spring into action in a fight-or-flight fashion. The parasympathetic system, on the other hand, has a different job. It's responsible for slowing your heartbeat, allowing your blood vessels to dilate and improving blood flow.

High heart rate variability generally indicates good health, while too little variability has been linked to a higher risk of disease. Researchers think that this may be because lower variability may allow more inflammation in the body, which can lead to disease.

When you have a good balance with your parasympathetic system, there's more variability because one system is urging the heart to beat faster, while the other is working to slow it down. Higher variability means there's a more active balance between the two systems, and this has been shown to improve health.

True or false? There's nothing you can do to improve your heart rate variability.
Answer: False.
When you're faced with stress, it's appropriate for the sympathetic system to kick in and release the hormones necessary for you to react to the stressor. But long-term, constant stress causes this reaction to be turned on too often. When the sympathetic system is triggered too often on a long-term basis, more stress hormones than are necessary course through the body. In turn, the parasympathetic system kicks in to try to help relieve the sympathetic system. When both of these parts of your autonomic nervous system operate in overdrive like this on an ongoing basis, your heart rate variability is affected, and you're left feeling edgy, yet sluggish — and your risk of many different heart problems increases. The good news is, you can do something about this.

Meditation, for example, is one area researchers are studying in terms of ways you can reduce the activity of the sympathetic nervous system and increase that of the parasympathetic system. Doing this increases heart rate variability, which in turn is thought to help lower your risk of disease.

Deep breathing and relaxation are other ways you can improve your heart rate variability. The simple act of slowing your breathing from 12 to 14 times a minute — a typical, natural rhythm — down to five or six breaths a minute can increase the activity in your parasympathetic nervous system, producing a relaxation response throughout your body.

Rest and relaxation

Although rest and relaxation are among the best ways to manage stress, they often are forgotten even though they're as critical to good health as a nutritious diet and regular physical activity.

Rest and relaxation both help slow your heart rate, so your heart doesn't have to work as hard. Relaxation lowers blood pressure and increases blood flow to your major muscles. Rest — in terms of regular, deep sleep — can improve immune function and reduce signs and symptoms of illness, such as headaches, nausea and pain.

Benefits of rest and relaxation

Does each day arrive with a long list of tasks to accomplish, with rest and relaxation at the very end of the list — if it even makes it on the list at all? If you can relate to this, you are not alone.

Instead of keeping this pattern going, consider reversing the order of your to-do list. Set aside adequate time for sleep and relaxation and then see how many of the tasks on your list you can get done in the time you have remaining. You may be surprised. That's because rest and relaxation benefit your health in a number ways. They:

- Slow your heart rate, meaning less work for your heart
- Reduce your blood pressure
- Increase blood flow to your major muscles
- Slow your breathing rate
- Lessen muscle tension
- Reduce signs and symptoms of illness, such as headaches, nausea, diarrhea and pain
- Give you more energy
- Improve your concentration

Tips for a good night's sleep

Getting seven to eight hours of good-quality sleep each night offers many benefits to your overall wellness. It can give you more energy and improve your concentration during the day. A good night's sleep can even help you lose weight.

That's because when you're tired, you may eat more high-calorie foods to keep your energy up. But when you're well-rested, you don't need those calories to stay alert.

If you have trouble sleeping or if you want to improve how well you sleep, making simple changes in your daily routine may help. Try these self-care tips to get a good night's sleep and all of the benefits that good, regular sleep offers.

- **Develop and stick to a sleep routine.** Reading a book is how many people lull themselves to sleep. Some gentle tai chi may help you relax. Turn off the TV and all other electronic devices about an hour before bed. Go to bed and get up about the same time every day, including weekends.
- **Cut down on caffeine, especially in the hours before bedtime.** Nonherbal teas, iced tea, coffee and many soft drinks have caffeine. Even chocolate (especially dark chocolate) has some caffeine, so look for all sources. Keep in mind that if you're used to drinking a lot of caffeine and you cut back suddenly, you may have a headache or be unusually sleepy for a couple of days but you'll soon feel better, and your sleep quality will improve.
- **Exercise and stay active.** Physical activity enhances deep and refreshing sleep. But avoid exercising too close to bedtime. If you exercise too close to bedtime, you might be too ener- gized to fall asleep. If this seems to be an issue for you, exercise earlier in the day.
- **Don't go to bed either hungry or too full.** Your discomfort might keep you awake.
- **Avoid alcohol and nicotine before bed- time.** They both interfere with healthy sleep. If you're bothered by heartburn, don't eat for a few hours before you lie down.
- **Avoid 'trying to sleep' or worrying about not getting enough sleep.** Hide your alarm clock in a drawer or turn it away from you if you find yourself looking at it too often. If sleep doesn't come naturally, read a book or listen to music until you feel drowsy.
- **Create comfort. Keep your bedroom quiet, dark and comfortably cool.** If you need them, consider using room-darkening

shades, earplugs, a fan or other devices to create an environment that suits your needs.

- **Avoid or limit daytime naps.** Long naps can make it difficult to fall asleep at night. If you choose to nap during the day, limit yourself to about 10 to 30 minutes and make it during the midafternoon.
- **Check your medications.** Ask your doctor if any of your medications — prescription, nonprescription and supplements you may be taking — can contribute to insomnia. Many prescription drugs can interfere with sleep, and many over-the-counter medications contain caffeine and other stimulants.

If you're having trouble sleeping, don't ignore it. Long-term, chronic insomnia can increase your risk of depression and anxiety disorders and can make chronic conditions, such as high blood pressure and diabetes, more severe.

Integrative treatments for insomnia

Although both prescription and nonprescription medications can help you sleep, they generally aren't recommended for long-term use. But many complementary treatments are used to help treat insomnia. As with any integrative treatment you haven't used before, discuss the pros and cons of each with your health care team first to ensure that the treatment you'd like to try is safe and appropriate for you.

Melatonin. Melatonin is a hormone produced naturally in the brain, and although melatonin supplements are widely used for jet lag, sometimes people take them to help them sleep. Melatonin is widely considered safe, but it may cause clotting problems in people taking blood thinners such as warfarin (Coumadin). Don't take it if you're pregnant or trying to become pregnant.

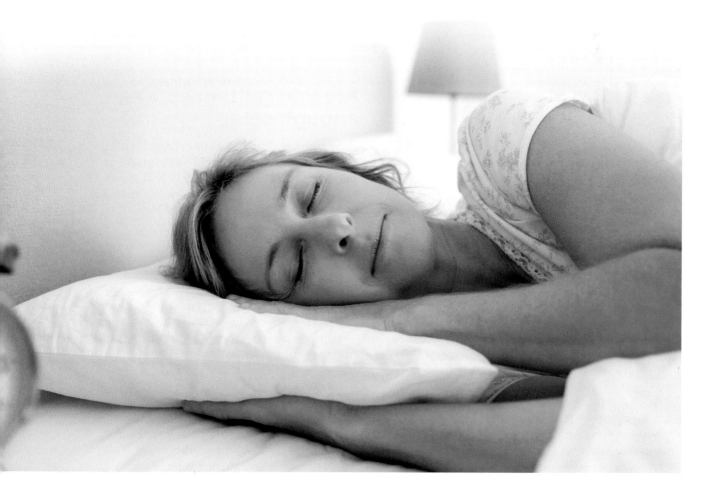

Valerian. The plant-based supplement valerian may help you get to sleep faster and improve sleep quality. Valerian is also used for anxiety. Research from a multicenter study found that a combination of valerian and hops may help treat insomnia. Discuss valerian with your doctor before trying it. Some people who have used high doses or used it long term may have increased their risk of liver damage, although it's not clear if valerian caused the damage.

Acupuncture and hypnosis. Acupuncture and hypnosis also are commonly used to help with insomnia, although researchers are unclear about their value.

Relaxation and wellness

Just as getting enough good-quality rest is essential to good health, so is relaxation. Together, rest and relaxation can make it easier for you to concentrate, improve your relationships with others and improve your productivity at work. You will learn later in this book about specific relaxation techniques. For now, let's focus on another important part of relaxation: leisure.

Find the right leisure activities

Leisure activities — what you choose to do during your free time — can reduce stress and improve your outlook on life.

More and more research shows that people who plan time for unwinding, visiting family and friends, playing sports, or taking part in religious activities have lower blood pressure and stress hormone levels. They are also more satisfied with their lives.

Leisure activities vary from person to person. What someone else finds interesting and pleasurable you may find boring or even stressful.

If you're in need of ideas for leisure activities, consider starting with your self-care needs. Answering these questions can help guide you in choosing fulfilling leisure activities.

- **Are you getting enough physical activity and exercise?** Regular physical activity promotes both physical and mental health.
- **Do you challenge yourself mentally?** It's important to do things that are mentally stimulating.
- **Are you meeting your spiritual needs?** Depending on how you define spirituality, you might take part in organized religious activities or express yourself through music or art, whether you're creating it or experiencing it.
- **Are you using your creative abilities?** What gets your creative juices flowing? Maybe it's dancing, painting, cooking or doing repair work on your house.
- **Do you have enough social contact with others?** If your answer is no, you might join a sports league or a book or dining club. Social interaction is an important part of wellness.
- **Is there novelty or adventure in your life?** Don't be afraid to experience new things. Consider traveling, hiking, or learning a new skill or hobby.
- **Are you interested in service to others?** If you like helping others, look for opportunities to volunteer.

Are you getting enough sleep?

Many people think they're getting adequate sleep but really aren't. You may not be getting the right amount and quality of sleep if you:

- Routinely ignore your alarm clock or catch a few extra minutes of sleep in the mornings
- Wake up groggy and don't feel refreshed
- Look forward to catching up on sleep on the weekends
- Are irritable with co-workers, family and friends
- Have difficulty concentrating or remembering
- Have to fight to stay awake during long meetings or after a meal
- Wake up repeatedly throughout the night

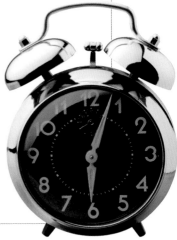

Connecting with others

Strong social ties are important to health and wellness because they're one component of living a purposeful life.

Benefits of relationships

Healthy relationships appear to boost your health in many ways. People in your social circle can:
- Help you celebrate good times and provide support during bad times
- Prevent loneliness and give you a chance to offer needed companionship
- Increase your sense of belonging and purpose
- Boost your happiness
- Lower your stress
- Improve your self-confidence and self-worth
- Help you cope with traumas, such as divorce, serious illness, job loss or a loved one's death
- Encourage you to change or avoid unhealthy lifestyle habits, such as excessive drinking or lack of exercise

Strengthening your relationships

Foster relationships with the people who are most important to you with these ideas, which come from Amit Sood, M.D., chair of the Mind Body Initiative within the Mayo Clinic Resilience program. (Learn more from Dr. Sood on page 39.)

Socialize at family gatherings

Sometimes, planning and preparing for gatherings becomes more important than the actual gathering itself. Take time to visit with others.

Eat together as a family

Family meals can help you influence children's behavior and development. Studies show that adolescents who share family meals have healthier eating habits and body weight, do better in school, have a better psychological well-being, and are less likely to get into drugs and alcohol or other trouble.

Be active together

Whether you go to community events or races, volunteer and give back to others, take a walk, or meet up at a park, get out and do something together. This gives you the chance to be active and enables you to have experiences and build good memories together.

Nurture friendships

Maintaining healthy relationships requires a little give and take. Try to respect your friends' boundaries, don't compete, and don't complain too much. Take a genuine interest in what's going on in your friends' lives, and don't judge them. Give your family and friends space to change, grow and make mistakes, and keep confidential any personal information that they share. Investing time in making friends and strengthening your friendships can pay off in better health.

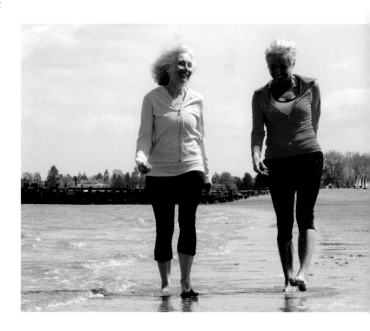

Mind-body techniques

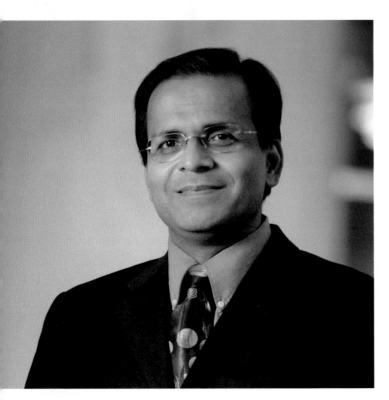

Amid Sood, M.D.
General Internal Medicine

Dr. Sood chairs the Mayo Mind-Body Initiative at Mayo Clinic in Rochester, Minnesota.

A visit with Dr. Sood

Years ago, if you said you wanted to take part in any type of mind-body medicine, the reaction you received may have been of concern — as though maybe you were weak or going through stress, because that seemed to be the only time that these types of practices came into play.

But today, taking a short meditation break, practicing deep breathing, or taking part in another type of mind-body medicine is more accepted. Mind-body practices have now come to the forefront of people's lives as a way to maintain health and wellness.

Every type of mind-body medicine, when tested, has been shown to offer benefits. So it doesn't matter what mind-body practice you choose, as long as it makes sense for you.

When I'm asked what is the best type of mind-body practice, I always suggest that people approach mind-body medicine as they do different aspects of life, such as a healthy diet, exercise or even relationships. Ask yourself three questions: First, *What are my beliefs?* Second, *What modalities are most accessible to me?* And finally, *What is practical?* The answers to these three questions will help you choose a practice that you can integrate into your life. For example, if you have just five or 10 minutes during the day, starting with a 45-minute meditation practice won't be practical for you. Likewise, don't choose a practice that doesn't align with your beliefs.

From a biological perspective, mind-body practices have distinct effects on the body that can help you live a longer, healthier, more enjoyable life. You'll read more about the effects of specific mind-body techniques in this section.

But mind-body practices have another benefit, as well, aside from their positive effects on your physical health. They can anchor you in intentional presence in a way that helps you feel less stressed and get more out of life.

What is mind-body medicine?

In today's world, people are often faced with health conditions, such as fibromyalgia and irritable bowel syndrome, that medication or surgery can't cure. This recognition — along with scientific evidence that the mind is one of several factors in the development of disease — has led to a renewed interest in the mind-body connection.

A two-way street

Research has shown that the mind can have a powerful influence on the body — but this connection is a two-way street. The body, and physical ailments that affect it, can significantly affect the mind. For example, people who have diabetes are two to three times more likely to be depressed, and people who have chronic pain often experience anxiety.

Just as your body can affect your mind, the mind can affect your body. That's why integrative medicine specialists believe that your mind and body must be in harmony for you to stay healthy. This is the premise behind *mind-body medicine*, which is designed to strengthen the communication between your mind and your body.

At its core, mind-body medicine focuses on how the power of your thought process can change what's happening in your body. You can't wish cancer away or think hard enough to make your diabetes disappear, but you can train your attention. And by training your attention, you can address anxiety and even create new pathways in your brain that help you experience less stress and anger.

Mind-body approaches aren't magic and they aren't a miracle cure, but with practice and patience, they do help. Mind-body medicine also offers you the opportunity to choose therapies that best fit your needs and style.

How the mind operates

To better understand mind-body medicine, it's helpful to know how the mind operates. This starts with two processes that take place at the same time in your mind. Together, they craft your everyday experiences. These processes are known as *attention* and *interpretation*.

Attention. The process of attention helps you screen, select and absorb sensory information from the world.

Interpretation. Your interpretation of the world around you depends on previous experience, preferences and how you planned for things to go. The lessons you learn through your experiences help you live an efficient and productive life. Although how you interpret the world helps you understand it and take action, interpretation can also have a downside: mindlessness.

Mindlessness

How you interpret the world is based on your preferences, prejudices and principles. They can lead you to make conclusions that are exaggerated and overgeneralized — and they can keep you from viewing the world around you in a way that encompasses the views and interests of others. In turn, you focus more time and effort on how you perceive the world around you rather than experiencing it for what it is. The way you attend to the world around you can lead to feelings of stress, which can lead to illness.

Simply put, if you are constantly **attending** to what's wrong in the world, or in yourself or in other people, you're **interpreting** your world in a mostly negative way.

When you're constantly attending to what's wrong in the world or in yourself, you're also likely to exaggerate those negative thoughts, so that small irritations become large threats, and you feel chronically anxious and stressed. You may develop a rigid outlook — *That won't work!* or, *That never happens!* This can get in the way of your ability to see things from a more mature perspective, which takes other viewpoints and outcomes into consideration. Mind-body therapists call this situation *mindlessness.*

In a state of mindlessness, you become disengaged from the real world and what it's really like. Instead, you ultimately focus mainly on thoughts that only make you feel anxious. A mindless state not only invites stress, sleeplessness and decreased quality of life, but also may increase your risk of multiple medical conditions, some of them potentially life-threatening.

How mind-body medicine can help

Mind-body techniques are designed to help free you from excessive negative thoughts and the related state of mindlessness. The idea is to develop a more-intentional focus. This, in turn, leads to a state of acceptance that empowers you to engage in meaningful action.

The idea behind mind-body medicine is to replace negative thoughts with a focus on principles such as forgiveness, acceptance, compassion, gratitude, interconnectedness and a higher meaning to life. These principles can help you see the reality — or lack thereof — in your thoughts.

The mind-body connection

Mind-body medicine is based on the idea that a combination of mental and emotional factors regulate physical health and that behavioral, psychological, social and spiritual techniques can enhance the mind's capacity to affect the body. The belief that mind and body are intricately connected goes back centuries.

How mind-body practices work

Mind-body practices have two core components.

Peaceful neutrality
The first step in mind-body medicine is to restore the mind to a state of peaceful neutrality. This means that the mind achieves a state that's nonjudgmental, efficient and adaptive to the needs of the individual.

To reach this state, the mind has to shed negative experiences acquired over the years.

Put your mind to work
The second step in mind-body medicine is to train your mind in a way that helps you achieve

beneficial health effects. You might use spiritual intervention (prayer), spoken intervention (transcendental meditation), or practices involving breathing and posture (yoga), or soothing imagery (guided imagery).

What the research says

Researchers have uncovered several ways in which the mind and body work together to achieve healing and enhance wellness. Here's a sampling of what researchers have learned about how the mind and body work together.

Stress response vs. relaxation response
The *stress response* is the fight-or-flight response — it automatically kicks in when you're faced with danger. Your body pumps up your heart rate, increases blood flow to your muscles and

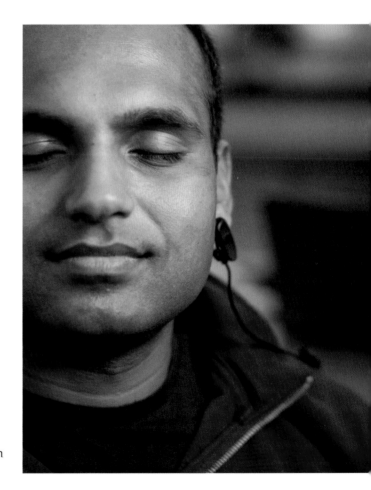

decreases blood flow to the parts of your body that aren't needed to face the threat.

The opposite of the stress response is the *relaxation response.* This is something that takes practice, but through approaches such as practicing meditation or deep breathing, you can train your body in a way that slows down your heart rate and your breathing and increases your focus on the present moment.

The way your mind can work in these two instances highlights the power of the mind-body connection — and makes mind-body medicine an ongoing area of medical study.

Can minds work together?

Researchers are also studying how mind and body respond to the healing effect of other minds. The positive benefits of interventions such as support groups may relate in part to the comfort and sense of security that comes with being part of a "tribe."

Studies in the last 20 or 30 years reaffirm the importance of the mind-body connection. Practitioners are using research findings to help people improve their health by recognizing how the mind and body affect each other.

Neuroplasticity

One final concept to keep in mind in terms of the mind-body connection is *neuroplasticity.* Neuroplasticity means that the brain is "plastic" or changeable, and that you can retrain it to react in more-skillful ways.

Retraining your brain

Neuroplasticity involves retraining the brain and involves attention and interpretation, which you learned about earlier in this section.

When you train your attention and interpretation, you're creating new ways of paying attention to the world around you and opening yourself up to new ways of thinking. For example, maybe that person who cut you off in traffic is on the way to the hospital to get to a loved one who's been in a tragic accident. With compassion in mind, how does your body react? Do you feel and react

differently knowing that information? Or do you still react with anger?

By creating new ways of thinking and using them again and again, you can reduce your stress and focus on principles — such as gratitude — that will help give your life deeper meaning.

What the research says

The concept of neuroplasticity is fairly new. Not that long ago, the general thinking was that the brain has a set number of neurons. The idea was that with age, not much good could happen to the neurons in the brain, but several bad things were likely, such as shrinkage of the brain, loss of those neural connections and, of course, conditions such as Alzheimer's disease.

However, research in the last 10 or 15 years has shown that the brain is not static. On the contrary, it has a great deal of neuroplasticity. You can create new connections in your brain at any age.

A healthy lifestyle matters

Healthy choices encourage neuroplasticity. A healthy diet that includes berries, getting regular aerobic exercise, connecting socially with others and creating novelty for your brain on a regular basis are all helpful.

Variety is key

For quite some time, mental exercises — working on crossword or jigsaw puzzles — were thought to help keep your brain active. But researchers have learned that variety is important, too. Just as you add variety to your physical activity to keep it interesting, research shows that it's important to vary the activities you do to keep your brain engaged, as well.

Once you start doing crossword puzzles, for example, your brain gets used to it, and it's no longer as challenging. So keep trying new activities. Learn a new language, try a new hobby — do something different to engage your brain.

Now that you understand a little more about mind-body medicine and how the mind works, let's turn to mind-body techniques that are proved to be useful in integrative medicine.

Relaxation therapies

Relaxation therapies involve refocusing your attention on something calming and increasing awareness of your body. They range from paced or deep breathing, to meditation and progressive muscle relaxation, and even art therapy and music therapy.

Some of the relaxation therapies you'll read about in this section take practice. As you learn these techniques, you'll become more aware of muscle tension and other physical sensations of stress. Once you know what the stress response feels like, you can make a conscious effort to practice a relaxation technique the moment you start to feel stress symptoms. This can prevent stress from spiraling out of control.

Before you start

For techniques that require practice, such as deep breathing and progressive muscle relaxation, it may take time for you to fully experience their benefits. Be patient with yourself. Don't let your effort to practice these techniques turn into one more source of stress.

If one relaxation technique doesn't work for you, try another. If none of your efforts at stress reduction seem to work, talk to your doctor about other options.

On the following pages, you'll read about five different types of relaxation therapies.

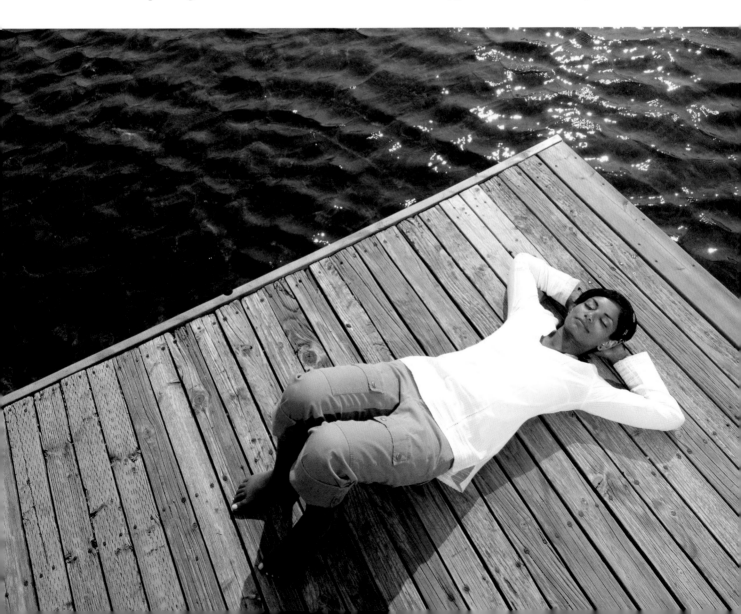

Progressive muscle relaxation

Progressive muscle relaxation is designed to reduce the tension in your muscles. It can be used to reduce anxiety and stress, which may be related to a medical condition. Or, progressive muscle relaxation may also be used simply to improve concentration.

Progressive muscle relaxation is a technique that focuses on the slow, steady shortening or tensing of a muscle, followed by a gradual relaxation phase in which you lengthen and release the muscle. The process is then repeated on other groups of muscles in succession.

In meditation, the idea is to try to get the body as still and quiet as possible. (Learn about meditation on page 56.) Progressive muscle relaxation is similar to meditation in that the goal is to try to reach a state of deep relaxation. However, progressive muscle relaxation differs from meditation in that relaxation is achieved through tensing and then relaxing various muscle groups in sequence.

By tensing and relaxing various muscle groups in sequence, you learn to identify areas in which extra stress or tension is being stored in your muscles and then deliberately relieve that tension.

Anyone experiencing stress can benefit from progressive muscle relaxation. This technique can be especially helpful for people who are new to meditation or other relaxation strategies.

There are no licensing or certification requirements for teaching progressive muscle relaxation, but many health care professionals have received training as part of their formal education.

Many cancer hospitals and clinics offer relaxation training programs that include progressive muscle relaxation. Your health care team may be able to recommend one for you to try.

How to do it

Try progressive muscle relaxation by taking these two steps.

Step 1
Beginning with your face, tighten the muscles around your eyes, nose and mouth so that you form a tight grimace. Hold the tension to the count of eight, exhale, and then allow your entire face to become loose and free. You're bringing oxygen to those tight muscles and then when you let go, the muscles relax.

Step 2
Move down the body, completely tensing your neck, then your jaw and then your shoulders, holding each set of muscles for eight seconds and then releasing them. Continue in your chest, abdomen, arms, hands, fingers, buttocks, legs, feet and toes until all of your muscle groups have been contracted and relaxed.

If you don't have much time, you can still use progressive muscle relaxation by targeting just a few areas, such as your face and neck, arms, shoulders and abdomen, chest and buttocks, legs and feet. Your larger muscle areas are contracted at once, rather than in smaller groups of muscles. The effect may feel like the gentle unraveling of a tightly sprung coil.

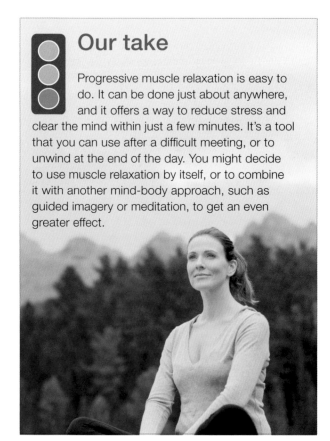

Our take

Progressive muscle relaxation is easy to do. It can be done just about anywhere, and it offers a way to reduce stress and clear the mind within just a few minutes. It's a tool that you can use after a difficult meeting, or to unwind at the end of the day. You might decide to use muscle relaxation by itself, or to combine it with another mind-body approach, such as guided imagery or meditation, to get an even greater effect.

What the research says

A growing body of evidence supports the effectiveness of progressive muscle relaxation in the treatment of certain conditions.

Although there haven't been many major studies focused on progressive muscle relaxation, research that has been done shows that it seems to help people of many ages with many different types of concerns. Here are some examples.

Anxiety and stress

In a small study years ago, 10 women between 60 and 84 years old who had lost their husbands within the past five years took part in a five-month progressive relaxation study. The women all reported feeling anxious and tense. After 10 weeks of practicing progressive relaxation, the women all said they felt less anxious.

Headache

Some studies have shown promising results when relaxation techniques have been used to reduce the symptoms of tension headache. For example, in the study of 10 women listed in the anxiety and stress section above, participants in the study experienced improvements in their headaches after practicing progressive muscle relaxation for 10 weeks.

In another study, people who had migraine headaches had significantly fewer migraine headaches after being trained in progressive muscle relaxation.

Finally, researchers studied about 90 people who had migraine or tension-type headaches. They found that 10 weeks of treatment that included progressive muscle relaxation, as well as education in how to set goals and in coping strategies for pain and stress, was a helpful addition to standard medical care in managing headache pain.

High blood pressure

In several clinical studies, relaxation techniques have been shown to lower blood pressure in people with hypertension.

However, although these studies are promising, it's important to know that the studies that have been conducted have used different types of relaxation therapies, and in most of the research, relaxation techniques were paired with other therapies. This makes it difficult to say with certainty how helpful relaxation techniques truly are in terms of lowering blood pressure.

With all of this said, researchers do say that progressive muscle relaxation is linked to a reduction in blood pressure.

Sleep

In the same small study referred to in the anxiety and stress section, women between ages 60 and 84 years old who had lost their husbands were able to fall asleep and stay asleep more easily after taking part in a five-month progressive relaxation program.

Stress

In a study conducted several years ago, about 70 men were exposed to a stressful situation.

The researchers separated the men into four groups and asked each group to do something different.

- One group was asked to listen to classical music.
- Another group was asked to listen to a story and write down what they heard.
- A third group was asked to sit in silence.
- Another group was asked to practice progressive muscle relaxation.

The men who completed progressive relaxation exercises were the most relaxed of all of the men in the study and felt the least amount of tension. The men who practiced progressive muscle relaxation also had a lower level of the stress hormone cortisol in their systems.

Cancer

Breast cancer has been a focus of research in the use of progressive muscle relaxation. Studies of women with breast cancer show that progressive muscle relaxation can help:

- Reduce nausea, vomiting, anxiety and depression
- Improve quality of life
- Reduce how long women have to stay in the hospital after undergoing a radical mastectomy

Deep breathing

Breathing is a fairly straightforward process: You take in oxygen and release carbon dioxide. Your chest rises and falls, because you likely breathe mostly through your chest — even though this isn't the most efficient way to breathe.

Deep, or relaxed, breathing is a technique that helps you breathe more efficiently. It involves deep, even-paced breathing using your diaphragm — the muscle under your rib cage — to expand your lungs. That's why this technique is also sometimes called *diaphragmatic breathing* or *paced breathing*. The purpose of deep breathing is to slow your breathing, take in more oxygen and reduce the use of shoulder, neck and upper chest muscles while you breathe.

When you practice deep breathing, you take a deep breath of air, pause, exhale and then pause before repeating. Your breaths are slow, smooth and deep.

Effects of deep breathing

Practicing deep breathing causes several effects in your body. Deep breathing:
- Releases your body's natural painkillers, feel-good chemicals called *endorphins*
- Increases blood flow to your major muscles
- Makes it easier for your heart to do its work
- Relaxes muscles that have been bracing against pain you have been feeling
- Helps your body and mind relax and regain strength and energy
- Helps you relax by reducing stress chemicals in your brain
- Provides a focus for your mind, which means less opportunity to think about stressful things

Safety

Deep breathing is a generally safe mind-body approach, but you may want to avoid it if you experience dizziness or tend to hyperventilate. Dizziness, tingling in your extremities and fainting are all possible on rare occasion with deep breathing.

How to do it

To get started with deep breathing, here are some general instructions to follow.
- First, lie on your back or sit comfortably with your feet flat on the floor.
- Next, relax your shoulders as you breathe.
- Then, breathe in slowly through your nose, allowing your abdomen to expand. Your chest should move only slightly.
- Finally, breathe out slowly through your mouth. Repeat this sequence as many times as you like.

Our take

As with other relaxation techniques, deep breathing is easy to do, it can be done just about anywhere, and it's an easy way to reduce stress and anxiety without any expense.

Deep breathing can be learned through formal instruction, or you can follow the simple instructions on this page to get started. As with other mind-body therapies, relaxed breathing may be combined with guided imagery or meditation. There's little risk in giving it a try.

What the research says

There's evidence that deep breathing can help treat several diseases and conditions.

Chronic obstructive pulmonary disease (COPD)

Altered breathing and shortness of breath are common in people who have chronic obstructive pulmonary disease (COPD). Although deep breathing doesn't seem to have any additional benefit when it's added to physical exercise, deep breathing has been shown to help people who have COPD walk farther. Other research shows that deep-breathing exercises can help improve quality of life for people who have COPD.

Chronic pain

Deep breathing is known for its chronic pain-relieving qualities. Researchers have found that deep breathing is one of many integrative techniques that are effective in helping manage several types of chronic pain. For example, studies on neck pain show that stress management techniques, including deep breathing, are a simple, no-cost way to manage stress that can cause neck pain.

Hot flashes

Some evidence shows that deep breathing can help reduce hot flashes that come with menopause, including how often they occur and how severe they are. In a study of about 70 women, those who used an audio CD to practice deep breathing once or twice a day had fewer hot flashes. The women also said that taking six breaths a minute for 15 minutes once or twice a day was something they could easily do on most days.

Nausea and vomiting

People who are prone to motion sickness have been able to reduce their symptoms of nausea by practicing deep breathing.

Asthma

Research shows that deep breathing improves quality of life in people who have asthma.

Insomnia

Tense muscles and anxiety are two causes of sleeplessness. Relaxation, on the other hand, has been shown to decrease wakefulness during sleep, making techniques such as deep breathing helpful. Several studies show that slow, paced breathing can help improve sleep quality.

Blood pressure

Deep breathing can help lower blood pressure. In one study of about 50 adults, researchers found that step-wise paced breathing, a breathing exercise in which you gradually reduce the number of breaths you take in a minute, significantly lowered blood pressure.

Anxiety and stress

Deep breathing can help decrease anxiety. Four randomized controlled trials and one study of slow-paced breathing were shown to help reduce symptoms of stress, anxiety, anger, exhaustion and depression, as well as improve quality of life.

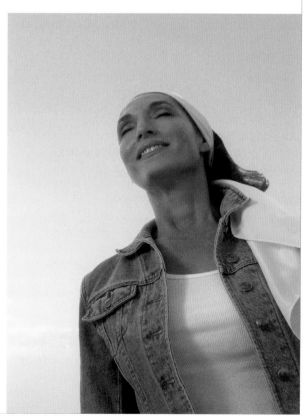

Art therapy

Art therapy involves the use of drawing, painting, sculpture and other art forms to allow expression and organization of your inner thoughts and emotions when talking about them is difficult. The creation of art itself, or interpretation of an art piece, is thought to be therapeutic. Self-expression through art therapy can help you cope with anxiety, stress, depression, and other mental and emotional issues.

The uses for art therapy range from helping war veterans, people who have anorexia, and people who have experienced abuse or trauma. Art therapy is practiced in a variety of settings, including hospitals, psychiatric and rehab facilities, wellness centers, schools, crisis centers, senior communities, private practice, and other clinical and community settings, in both individual and group sessions.

Art therapy can take many forms, from drawing and painting to pottery and card-making. Getting your hands into finger paint or modeling clay can release pent-up tension and get you in touch with deeper feelings. There are even coloring books and patterns specifically designed to help with anxiety, where people work with repetitive patterns to help break a panic cycle.

Torn paper collage

One example of an art therapy project that can help you cope with stress is called the "torn paper" collage. This technique can be helpful during times when you feel that the stress in your life is out of your control.

This technique allows you to take charge through the use of art materials. This exercise isn't about perfection, but rather just enjoying the process of tearing and constructing imagery. Here's how it works.

Step 1
Start with a variety of colored paper — even old scraps of wrapping paper that you have around the house, scraps of construction paper or pieces of colored newspaper. Tear the paper into shapes that appeal to you or use scissors to cut out pieces like tiles for more of a mosaic effect.

Step 2
Arrange the pieces carefully with a certain amount of space in between and get a tiled effect or the effect you would have putting together a puzzle. Or, arrange the shapes randomly on a page to make an interesting pattern.

Step 3
Once you place the pieces where you want them, use white glue or a glue stick and begin to glue your shapes down. From there, you can add pieces of paper, building around the pieces as you glue them. Whether you choose a planned pattern or work abstractly, you're making all of the choices, which helps reduce stress.

The torn paper collage exercise isn't about perfection, but rather just enjoying the process of tearing and constructing imagery.

 Our take

Although there haven't been many studies done on art therapy, those that have been done support the idea that artistic expression of any type can help you cope with day-to-day stress as well as a host of mental and emotional issues, including anxiety and depression.

What the research says

Alzheimer's disease

A 2014 review of research studies focused on the use of art therapy for Alzheimer's disease concluded that art therapy:

- Engages attention
- Provides pleasure
- Improves neuropsychiatric symptoms, social behavior and self-esteem

Other applications

Although more and larger studies are needed, several small studies show that art therapy shows promise in treating:

- Cancer
- Parkinson's disease
- HIV/AIDS
- Diabetes
- Stroke

In addition, numerous case studies demonstrate that art therapy offers benefits for people with both emotional and physical illnesses. Case studies of young people have involved burn recovery, eating disorders and sexual abuse. Studies of adults using art therapy have included bereavement, addictions and bone marrow transplants.

Art therapy at Mayo Clinic

Research conducted at Mayo Clinic shows that art therapy offers benefits to patients and staff alike.

For example, a small Mayo Clinic study involved an artist from the community who came to the bedside of very ill patients struggling with blood-based cancers.

In this particular study, the artist came to the bedside with a number of different media and then asked patients to choose a type of art therapy. Many of the people in the study said that they had no artistic talent, but nearly all of them found a way to express themselves using the various materials provided. In the process, the experience helped reduce participants' stress and pain, as well as improve their quality of life. Among their reactions to experiencing art therapy, study participants said:

- "It made me forget all my problems and think about other things totally unrelated to medical problems."
- "It was very enjoyable and lifted my spirits quite a bit."
- "This experience was very lovely. Keeping one's mind on things such as art is very inspiring."
- "Excellent way to remind the patient they are still alive … Yes you are a person."

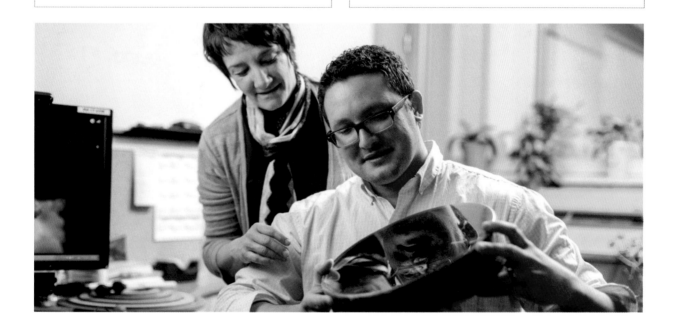

Music therapy

Similar to art therapy, music therapy is based on the belief that the creative process involved in artistic self-expression can help people resolve conflicts and problems and reduce stress.

Music therapy can enhance mood, promote relaxation and reduce anxiety. Playing of music — even during medical procedures — has also been shown to produce relaxing and calming effects.

How it works

Music therapy is different from listening to music. With music therapy, a trained music therapist works with a patient's health care team to come up with a plan that uses music therapy to meet the patient's specific needs. Music therapy can involve creating, singing, moving to and listening to music.

A music therapist is trained to assess a patient's strengths and needs and uses a variety of tools, music and instruments to help meet the patient's clinical goals.

Music therapy also provides avenues for communication that can be helpful to those who find it hard to express themselves in words. For example, music therapists worked with United States Congresswoman Gabby Giffords to help her regain her speech after surviving a bullet wound to the head.

Use of technology

While listening to a live performance in a hospital room can offer benefits, it isn't practical to always use live musicians for music therapy. With this in mind, researchers continue to study the role that technology plays in music therapy.

Because live music isn't always feasible to offer in music therapy, recorded music is used most often when music therapy is part of a patient's care. To date, studies conducted on music therapy seem to suggest excellent outcomes even when the music is recorded.

Our take

For many people, music occupies a central role in their lives. It revives their spirits, gets them moving and, in some cases, eases pain and suffering. Whether you listen to music simply for the joy and comfort that it brings, or you actively work with a trained music therapist as part of an overall treatment plan, music can be an important part of the healing process. There's scientific evidence that structured music therapy is effective in treating a number of conditions and disorders. Music therapy is sometimes combined with other approaches, including guided imagery, to achieve desired treatment goals.

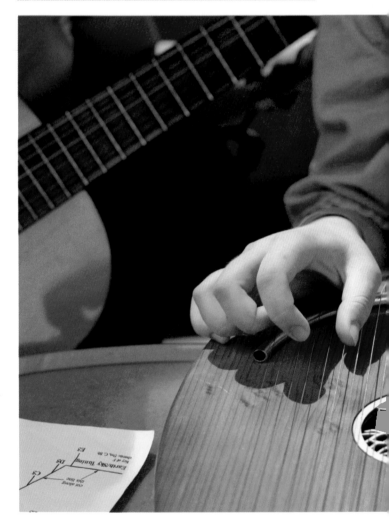

What the research says

Dementia

A 2015 meta-analysis found that music therapy improves disruptive behavior and reduces anxiety in people with dementia. In a small study of adults with Alzheimer's disease, two dozen sessions of music therapy involving singing that took place over six months improved behavioral and psychological symptoms of dementia. In general, listening to their favorite songs may help people with Alzheimer's disease feel calmer and less anxious.

Asthma

Two randomized controlled trials showed that playing a brass or wind instrument led to a decrease in asthma symptoms. In addition, music therapy improved mood and decreased depression and anxiety in people with asthma. A study of 76 adults with asthma showed that music therapy is a relaxation technique that can help improve lung function in people with mild asthma and reduce shortness of breath, especially in men.

Pain

In a controlled trial of 87 people with low back pain, fibromyalgia, inflammatory disease or neurological disease, two or more sessions of listening to music, along with standard treatment, led to a bigger reduction in pain when compared to people who did not listen to music. This effect lasted up to a month after the music therapy program ended. Listening to music also helped improve anxiety and depression, and reduce use of medication. Similar results were seen in another study that focused specifically on fibromyalgia.

Autism

Music therapy uses musical experiences to help people communicate and express their feelings — two of the core issues people with autism face. It's also been shown that children with autism tend to respond better to music than they do to spoken words. With these ideas in mind, researchers are studying how people with autism understand and more effectively express their feelings in words. Music is predictable, structured and success-oriented, and offers a sense of security, helping people interact more spontaneously with others. One small study of children with autism showed that music therapy can help improve social skills. The researchers noted that music therapy encourages children to establish relationships with others and better understand how other people feel. In another review, this time of 10 studies, researchers found that music therapy can help children with autism improve how well they interact and communicate with others.

Parkinson's disease

Music therapy can help people who have Parkinson's disease improve their motor skills. Researchers have found that music can help with some of the side effects typical of the disease — shuffling gait, tremors, rigid muscles and changes in speech. The idea here is that rhythm, like the beat of a drum or the tick of a metronome, can foster slow, coordinated movement when people try to move with the music. Singing exercises and playing kazoos also provide benefit by helping with breath support.

Mood enhancement

A 2015 study of 15 women receiving chemotherapy for breast cancer found that those who took part in mindfulness-based music therapy for one hour a week for four weeks experienced improvements in their mood. These women also felt that they could focus their attention better and felt less tired. Other research from 2015, this time a review of 25 studies, showed that music therapy improved mood, as well as depressive syndromes and quality of life in people with neurological disorders including stroke, epilepsy, multiple sclerosis and Parkinson's disease.

Relaxation and stress reduction

Researchers measuring the effects of stress — blood pressure, pulse, nervous system activity and feelings of stress — found that listening to music for 20 minutes has a positive, stress-reducing effect on the body. In a study of 64 college students, blood pressure, pulse and other effects on the body caused by stress were all improved after they listened to music for 20 minutes.

Animal-assisted therapy

Imagine you're in the hospital, and your doctor mentions that a therapy dog will be coming in to see patients who would like a visit. Your doctor asks if you would be interested in a visit, and you say yes.

Later in the day, a friendly therapy dog and his handler appear in your doorway, and with a gentle smile, the handler introduces them and says that they're there to visit you, so you invite them in.

You haven't been feeling well, but in a short time, as you stroke the dog's fur and get to know more about him from his handler, the pain and anxiety you've been feeling seem to disappear.

After the visit, you realize you're smiling. And you feel a little less tired and a bit more optimistic. You can't wait to tell your family all about the charming canine you met. In fact, you're already looking forward to the dog's next visit.

As you might imagine from this example, animal-assisted therapy offers a variety of benefits. It can significantly reduce pain, anxiety, depression and fatigue for:

- Children having dental procedures
- People receiving cancer treatment
- Residents in long-term care facilities
- People hospitalized with chronic heart failure
- Veterans with post-traumatic stress disorder

In some cases, these animals can also help with physical rehabilitation through activities such as throwing a ball or walking. Animal-assisted therapy is also used in nonmedical settings, such as universities and community programs, to help people manage anxiety and stress.

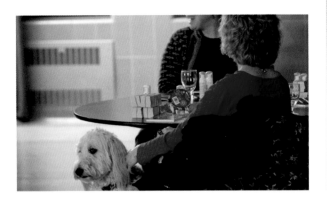

Our take

Animal-assisted therapy gets a green light when properly trained animals are used and certain rules regarding safety and sanitation are followed. Most hospitals and other facilities that use animal-assisted therapy have stringent rules to ensure that the animals are clean, vaccinated, well-trained and screened for appropriate behavior. It's also important to note that the Centers for Disease Control and Prevention has never received a report of infection from animal-assisted therapy.

However, animal-assisted therapy isn't suitable for everyone. For example, animal-assisted therapy isn't a good fit when someone's immune system is suppressed, or when a person simply doesn't enjoy visiting with a dog.

What the research says

Although the benefits of the bonds between humans and animals have been known for centuries, scientific research involving human-animal interactions has only been recorded since the 1960s.

Of the studies that have been conducted, research shows that animals can provide healing on a number of different levels. Here's what several studies show.

- Interacting with an animal can reduce anxiety, depression and loneliness, as well as improve social support and general well-being.
- Companion animals can contribute to recovery from a serious condition.
- Pet ownership has been shown to reduce heart rate, blood pressure, and triglyceride and cholesterol levels.
- Pets have been shown to help people cope with chronic conditions and illnesses, including heart disease, dementia and cancer, as well as developmental disabilities and mental health disorders, including depression, anxiety, attention deficit hyperactivity disorder and schizophrenia.

Animal-assisted therapy at Mayo Clinic

You might say that Mayo Clinic has gone to the dogs — but that's not a bad thing.

That's because on Mayo Clinic's Rochester, Arizona and Florida campuses, as many as 100 dogs are providing comfort to those in need as part of the Caring Canines animal-assisted therapy program. Therapy dogs in the Caring Canines program bring comfort to those in need. Animal-assisted therapy is a growing field, and it's one more type of relaxation therapy offered at Mayo Clinic.

Depending on whom you ask, you may hear visits from therapy dogs described as animal-assisted activities, animal-assisted therapy, animal-assisted interactions or even more simply as pet therapy. All of these terms have a similar definition: Specially trained dogs that provide comfort and a needed, positive distraction for people in need — including patients and their families, as well as staff, at Mayo Clinic.

What is Caring Canines?

Caring Canines is a group of Mayo Clinic volunteers who have been registered with their dogs through a nationally accredited organization that educates and evaluates therapy dog teams.

Along with their human volunteers, therapy dogs in the Caring Canines program:

- Offer compassion
- Support patients socially, physically and mentally
- Help motivate patients as part of their treatment
- Relieve anxiety
- Provide a distraction from illness

Of their many healing powers, Mayo Clinic's therapy dogs have the power to soothe stress and boost morale for anyone who crosses their paths.

Mayo Clinic has offered the Caring Canines program since 2002 in Rochester, and since 2011 in Arizona and Florida.

Where do Mayo Clinic therapy dogs visit?

According to Jessica Smidt, who heads Mayo Clinic's Caring Canines program in Rochester, Minnesota, there are very few places they *can't* go.

You may find Caring Canines teams visiting patients, their families, staff and visitors in:

- Outpatient waiting rooms
- Hospitals
- Psychology and psychiatry areas
- Physical therapy settings

Caring Canines teams are featured as part of structured group visits and also go door to door to see patients.

"We go around and bring comfort and joy to patients and take their minds off of being stuck in the hospital," Smidt says.

But that's not all — therapy dogs make the rounds at staff wellness events and even visit students to provide stress relief during midterms and finals.

Ensuring safety and sanitation

Animal-assisted therapy isn't for everybody, and important steps must be taken to ensure that it's safe for everyone involved. The biggest concern, particularly in hospitals, is safety and sanitation. Most hospitals and other facilities that use animal-assisted therapy have stringent rules to ensure that the animals are clean, vaccinated, well-trained and screened for appropriate behavior. But for those who are a good fit for receiving a visit from a therapy dog, the results can be miraculous for everyone involved.

"Almost every day, I'll have someone who will cry on Alta and say, 'This is the best part of my day,' and it literally brings tears to their eyes," Smidt says of her experiences with Alta, a facility-based service dog who partners with Smidt as part of the Caring Canines program.

In one instance, Smidt shared, a young girl was depressed and wouldn't come out of her hospital room. So a child life specialist contacted Smidt and asked her if she would bring Alta to an activity room to see if it would motivate the young girl to leave her room. Although it took some time, the girl eventually came to the room, snuggled up with Alta, and started to brighten up and talk with her doctor and her family.

"Everybody, even her mom, said, 'This is amazing. We've been waiting for this for days,'" Smidt said. "There's just something that everyone connects to with a dog. It's hard to explain why, but it's kind of like an innate connection."

Are you interested in volunteering with your dog?

If you're interested in volunteering as an animal-assisted therapy team with your dog, Jessica Smidt, who heads Mayo Clinic's Caring Canines program in Rochester, Minnesota, offers this advice:

Evaluate your dog. Where does your dog enjoy going? Does your dog truly enjoy going to different places and visiting with people?

"The best therapy dogs in our program are the ones that were born with the natural disposition to truly love everybody, aren't easily stressed, and are calm and mild-mannered," Smidt says.

Assess your dog's comfort level. Evaluate your dog to make sure that he or she is truly comfortable and happy visiting with strangers in unfamiliar environments.

Ask yourself if your dog:
- Is friendly and well-mannered
- Listens to your commands at all times
- Is predictable, reliable and controllable
- Is comfortable being touched, awkwardly at times
- Is comfortable being crowded by people

Take a class. Take any kind of all-positive, rewards-based class with your dog. Talk to the trainer to get another opinion of your dog's disposition, behavior and obedience level to see if your dog is a good fit for therapy work.

Think about where you would like to visit. If you have a facility in mind where you would like to visit with your dog, call and ask if the facility has any special requirements, including registration through a specific therapy dog organization.

Choose a reputable organization that tests and registers therapy dog teams. Facilities vary in terms of what therapy dog registration they prefer. If the location where you would like to visit doesn't prefer that you register as a therapy dog team with a specific organization, do your homework and choose the organization that fits you best. Three well-known national therapy dog registries are:

Alliance of Therapy Dogs – www.therapydogs.com
Pet Partners – https://petpartners.org
Therapy Dogs International – http://tdi-dog.org

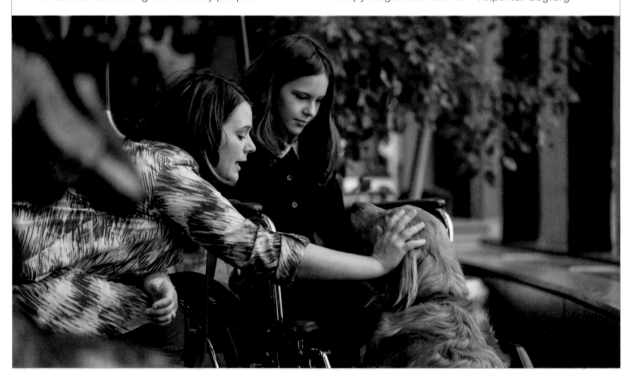

Expert insight
The power of the human-animal bond

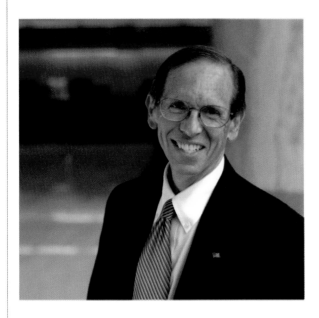

Edward T. Creagan, M.D.
Medical Oncology, Mayo Clinic, Rochester, Minnesota

Board-certified in hospice and palliative medicine, Dr. Creagan has authored several papers and given several presentations on the human-animal bond. He has witnessed firsthand the significant role that companion animals play in people's lives.

Every day, I visit with patients who are expected to live no more than 24 weeks. And every day, I'm faced with these kinds of questions: "Doc, is this my last Christmas?" or, "My daughter's wedding is in three months. Will I still be here? Should we move it up?"

These are tough, emotional questions to sort through — issues that many types of integrative medicine, including a bond with an animal, can help address.

In the United States, nearly three out of every four households has at least one pet. So it likely comes as no surprise that in the last 10 years, the amount of money spent on pets in the United States has nearly doubled. As the amount of time and money spent on companion animals increases, so does our knowledge about how pets can improve health, well-being and quality of life.

A pet can save your life

When you pet a dog or a cat or otherwise engage with an animal, you get a boost of "happy hormones" in your body, including oxytocin, serotonin and endorphins. This leads to a variety of health benefits.

- In a study of more than 300 people who were receiving chemotherapy to treat advanced cancer, those who had pets felt less stressed.
- Research suggests that animal-assisted therapy may help treat signs and symptoms of dementia.
- Elderly adults in nursing homes have better nutritional health when they eat their meals near an aquarium rather than eating alone.
- In a study of nearly 100 adults who had had a heart attack, almost two-thirds of those who survived a year afterward had pets.
- A 2013 statement from the American Heart Association cited 81 different studies showing that having a pet helps in managing high blood pressure, high cholesterol and obesity.

What these findings show can be put very simply: A pet can save your life.

In today's society, pets have become as important to families as humans. Domestic violence shelters are becoming pet-friendly. Hurricane Katrina changed how rescue organizations handle evacuations during natural disasters. It's becoming common practice for people to set aside money for the care of their pets and entrust someone with that responsibility, should they die and leave their pets behind.

At Mayo Clinic, we recognize how important companion animals are to patients, and as physicians, many of us add a pet's name to a patient's file. After we've talked about medical issues the patient is facing, we shift the conversation to the patient's pet. We find that taking time to talk to patients about their pets and to arrange for a patient's pet to be at the bedside at the end of life means more to patients and their families than I can ever put into words.

Meditation

The word *meditation* has become part of everyday vocabulary. You may hear people talking about meditating on television, sports figures saying they meditate as part of their exercise routine, and even some elementary schools incorporating meditation into their curriculums.

The term *meditation* refers to a group of techniques. Many meditation techniques have roots in Eastern religious or spiritual traditions, and some people consider praying a form of meditation. But like a lot of the mind-body practices you've learned about in this book, there's no one right way to meditate.

Meditation has been practiced for thousands of years. It originally was meant to help deepen understanding of the sacred aspects of life. In the 21st century, however, meditation has been considerably demystified.

No matter how you meditate, the goal is really the same: to focus your attention. Maybe your focus is on your breathing, as you inhale and exhale, or on a specific word that you're repeating. Or maybe you meditate by taking a moment of gratitude before you sit down at your desk.

The idea behind meditation is to suspend the stream of thoughts that normally occupies your conscious mind. Doing this leads to a state of physical relaxation, mental calmness and psychological balance.

Practicing meditation can change how you relate to the flow of your emotions and thoughts and it may help you control how you respond to a challenging situation. For example, if you're claustrophobic and you know you're going to have an MRI, meditating and focusing on your breathing as you inhale and exhale may help you feel less anxious and get through the exam. Or maybe public speaking makes you feel nervous. Taking five deep breaths before giving an important presentation may help you slow down, relax and focus.

Anyone can practice meditation. It's simple and inexpensive, and you don't need any special equipment to do it. In addition, meditation is a type of integrative medicine that you can practice wherever you are — whether you're out for a walk, riding the bus, waiting at the doctor's office or even in the middle of a tense business meeting.

Different types

If you're interested in starting a meditation practice, there are several options.

Analytical meditation

Analytical meditation involves focusing on an object and thinking about its deeper meaning. You might focus your attention on a scriptural passage or a concept, such as how precious human life is. The goal of this type of meditation is to focus on feeling empathy and compassion toward yourself and toward others.

Body scanning

Body scanning involves focused attention on different parts of your body. Through body scanning, you become aware of your body's various sensations, whether that's pain, tension, warmth or relaxation. You can combine body scanning with breathing exercises and imagine breathing heat or relaxation into and out of different parts of your body.

Breath meditation

This approach involves focusing on your breathing. It involves the conscious observing of every inhalation and exhalation, and the rising and

falling of the chest. Breathing that is deep, slow, diaphragmatic and smooth is maintained during this practice. The purpose is to slow your breathing, take in more oxygen, and reduce the use of shoulder, neck and upper chest muscles while breathing so that you breathe more efficiently.

Focus on love and gratitude

In this type of meditation, you focus your attention on a sacred object or being, weaving feelings of love, compassion and gratitude into your thoughts. You can also close your eyes and use your imagination or gaze at representations of the object of your focus.

Guided meditation

With guided meditation, you form mental images of places or situations you find relaxing. Try to use as many senses as possible, such as smells, sights, sounds and textures. You may be led through this process in a class by a guide or teacher, or you may prefer to use guided imagery programs on your own at home.

Mindfulness meditation

Mindfulness meditation is based on the concept of being mindful of — having an increased awareness and complete acceptance of — the present moment.

One mindful meditation exercise is to bring all your attention to the sensation of the flow of your breath in and out of your body. The goal is to focus on what's being experienced in the present, without reacting to it or making any judgments about it. This approach is used as a way of learning a more balanced response to the thoughts and emotions of daily life.

Transcendental meditation

In transcendental meditation, you focus on a mantra — a sound, word or phrase — repeated over and over, either out loud or to yourself. The goal is to keep distracting thoughts out of your conscious awareness.

You can create your own mantra, whether it's religious or secular. Examples of religious mantras include the Jesus Prayer in the Christian tradition, the holy name of God in Judaism, or the om mantra of Hinduism, Buddhism and other Eastern religions.

For a secular mantra, you can use the words *one*, *love* or *peace*, or any word or phrase that is meaningful to you. Whatever mantra you choose, it should hold your attention on a single thought or sensation that brings you a sense of comfort.

Walking meditation

This form of meditation — called *kinhin* in the Zen tradition — focuses on the subtle movements used to stand and walk. You focus your attention on the soles of your feet, first as you stand, and then as you walk.

Walking meditation requires that, for safety reasons, you pay greater attention to what's going on around you. You can use this technique anywhere you're walking, such as in a tranquil forest, on a city sidewalk or at the mall. When you use this method, keep these tips in mind:

- Slow down your pace so that you can focus on each movement of your legs or feet.
- Don't focus on a particular destination. Concentrate on your legs and feet, repeating action words in your mind such as *lifting*, *moving* and *placing* as you lift each foot; move your leg forward and place your foot on the ground.

Before you get started

There is no right way or wrong way to meditate. You can make meditation as formal or informal as you like, however it suits your lifestyle and situation. Some people build meditation into their daily routine — for example, starting and ending each day with time for meditation.

Other options include listening to sacred music, spoken words or any music you find relaxing or inspiring. You may want to write your reflections in a journal or discuss them with a friend or spiritual leader.

How meditation affects the body

Research shows that meditation offers several benefits. Here are several examples.

Meditation and emotional well-being

The purpose of meditation is to clear away the information overload that builds up every day and contributes to stress. The emotional benefits of meditation can include:

- Gaining a new perspective on stressful situations
- Building skills to manage your stress
- Increasing self-awareness
- Being able to focus on the present moment
- Reducing negative emotions
- Improving your memory and concentration
- Helping you stick to a physical activity program

Meditation and illness

Meditation may also be useful if you have a medical condition, especially one that may be worsened by stress. Research suggests that meditation can help people manage:

- Anxiety disorders
- Asthma
- Cancer
- Depression
- Heart disease
- High blood pressure
- Pain
- Sleep problems

Science supports many of these findings, as you'll learn on page 62. For example, Harvard researchers found that participating in an eight-week mindfulness meditation program appears to make measurable changes in the parts of the brain associated with memory, sense of self, empathy and stress. Researchers at UCLA have found that the brains of people who meditate were better preserved as they age when compared to the brains of people who don't meditate.

In some circumstances, it's clear that meditation is helpful, but it's not fully clear why. For example, in one study, researchers focused on the relationship between mindfulness meditation and its ability to reduce symptoms of depression, anxiety and pain. The researchers found that among people with depression, meditation produced a response similar to that of antidepressants. What's not fully clear yet is why.

How meditation works in the brain and the body

Practicing meditation has been shown to produce physical changes, such as in the body's fight-or-flight response to stress, which you read about earlier in this section. The system responsible for the fight-or-flight response is called the **autonomic nervous system** — sometimes also called the **involuntary nervous system**. It regulates many activities, including your heartbeat, blood pressure, perspiration, breathing rate, body temperature, the production of body fluids and digestion.

Research has also shown that meditation can be an effective way to slow the brain waves so you feel deeper relaxation. As each breath begins to lengthen, the brain waves begin to slow.

Building your skills

Meditation takes practice. As you practice your meditation skills, keep these points in mind:
- It's common for your mind to wander during meditation, no matter how long you've been practicing it.
- If you're meditating to calm your mind and your attention wanders, slowly return to the object, sensation or movement that you're focusing on.
- Experiment, and you'll likely find the types of meditation that work best for you and what types of meditation you enjoy doing most.
- Adapt meditation to your needs at the moment. Remember, there's no right way or wrong way to meditate.
- In the end, what matters most about meditation is that it helps you reduce your stress level and feel better overall.

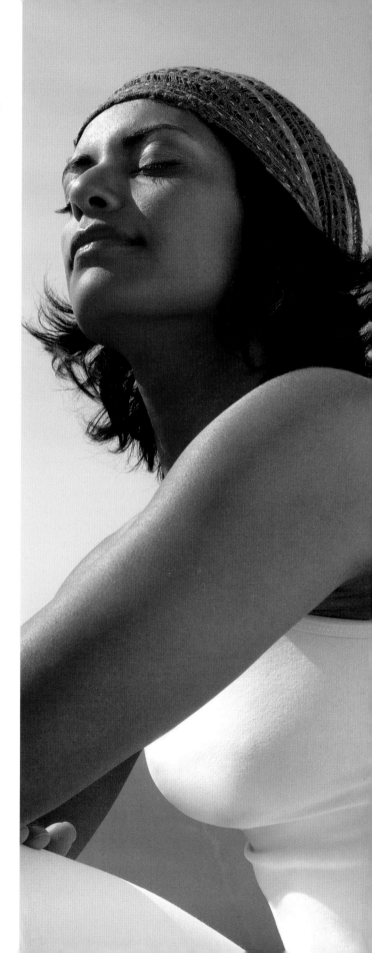

Getting ready

Most types of meditation require four elements.

1. A quiet place

Many people who meditate prefer a place with as few distractions as possible. This can be particularly helpful for those just starting to practice meditation.

2. A specific posture

Depending on the type of meditation, it can be done while sitting, standing, lying down, walking or in other positions. You may sit against a wall if that's comfortable for you. A favorite cushion or a certain chair are other options.

3. Focused attention

Focusing your attention is an important part of meditating. For example, you may focus on a mantra — a specific word or set of words. You may also choose to focus on your breathing, or on an object such as a candle or an image.

4. An open mind

Let distractions come and go without engaging them — without stopping to think about them. When distracting or wandering thoughts occur during meditation, gently bring your attention back to the focus. In some types of meditation, you may learn to observe the rising and the falling of thoughts and emotions as they occur.

Our take

Meditation may be the perfect complement to the rush of a busy, complicated life. As the evidence supporting the use of meditation grows, adding it to your daily schedule may be just the antidote you need to deal with a hectic routine. In addition, if meditation helps to lower your blood pressure and reduce stress in your life, so much the better. The long-term benefits of meditation continue to undergo study.

Meditation at Mayo Clinic

Nurses in Mayo Clinic's Healing Enhancement Program, known as *integrative therapy specialists*, may arrange for massage or a visit from a music therapist or a Caring Canines therapy dog team. But they can provide services on their own as well, including meditation.

Meditation at Mayo Clinic features a focus on its universal elements, including focused slowed breathing and focused attention. Making meditation a secular practice — while honoring its main components — has been a key strategy in making meditation available to anyone who wants to explore it. The benefits of meditation are universal, meaning that they don't have to include a specific religious connection.

Focused attention, an important part of meditation, can be learned at Mayo Clinic through the SMART program, developed by Mayo Clinic physician Amit Sood, M.D. You learned about the SMART program earlier in this book (see page 14). SMART stands for Stress Management And Resiliency Training. This structured program is scientifically proved to:

- Reduce stress and anxiety
- Increase well-being and resilience
- Enhance gratitude
- Improve mindfulness
- Boost happiness
- Promote positive health behaviors

Participants in the SMART program learn how to train their attention so that it's stronger, more focused in the present moment and more intentional. They learn to guide their thoughts based on higher principles rather than by prejudices, which you learned about earlier in this section. The SMART program has been tested in 20 completed research studies in and outside of Mayo Clinic, all with positive results including those listed above.

Mayo Clinic's integrative medicine program also offers a meditation course for employees and patients. Participants in this course receive a DVD to practice meditation on their own. This course has been tested and shown to decrease anxiety and stress, as well as improve overall quality of life.

Expert insight

Dr. Bauer shares his experience with meditation

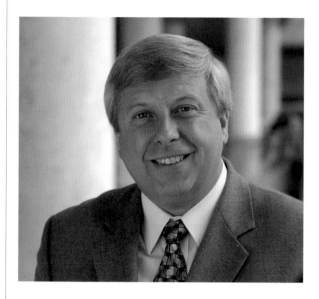

Brent A. Bauer, M.D.
Medical editor, *Mayo Clinic Guide to Integrative Medicine*

In addition to his role as a medical editor of this book, Dr. Bauer is director of research in Integrative Medicine and Health at Mayo Clinic in Rochester, Minnesota.

When I founded Mayo Clinic's integrative medicine program, I was convinced of the importance of meditation and tried to get patients to carve out 30 or even 60 minutes of time each day to meditate. This approach was not successful. People just didn't have that kind of patience. When Amit Sood, M.D. — whom you've heard from in this section — joined Mayo Clinic, he introduced the idea of meditating by doing simple things throughout the day.

Instead of carving out 30 minutes for meditation, maybe you do 15 minutes of meditation in the morning and then some guided imagery at night. Or you can try a simpler approach. Here are two examples Dr. Sood recommends:
1. When you wake up in the morning, think about five things or people you are grateful for.

2. Silently think, "I wish you well" to people you encounter throughout the day.

One of the things Dr. Sood taught me, personally, was to pause before I go into a patient's room, take three deep breaths and have kind intentions before I go in, even if I don't know the patient.

Advice on starting a meditation practice

When I talk with patients, I try to emphasize that it's OK to try different meditation practices. I don't want people to feel bad because they weren't able to sit and meditate for an hour. If one kind of meditation doesn't work for you, try something else that may be more your speed — maybe it's tai chi or yoga or going for a quiet walk. Whatever you can do to try to quiet your mind and let the thoughts flow by, that's what works for you.

It's also OK to meditate in the way that works best for you. Being physically still — actually sitting still — can be challenging. You might feel an itch, your back may hurt, your muscles may cramp or you may get fidgety. That's all OK.

Sometimes patients tell me they're worried that if they try to sit still and meditate, they'll fail. For these individuals, meditation was one more thing they felt bad about not doing. For some people, it's really a struggle to keep very quiet, and they get frustrated and think they're not doing it right. I encourage these individuals to try different practices until they find one that works for them.

Maybe sitting for 15 minutes in silence is a long-range goal, and that's OK. What's important is to start somewhere, no matter where it is, doing something that works for you.

If sitting in silence for 15 minutes doesn't work for you right now, maybe a practice that makes more sense for you is to focus on compassionate thoughts or kind intentions. In these cases, you're not sitting down to meditate; instead, you're being mindful toward the people you meet. That's meditation, too. Ultimately, what's important to remember is that any meditation is good meditation.

What the research says

Although a growing body of scientific research supports the health benefits of meditation, some researchers believe it's not yet possible to draw conclusions on this type of integrative therapy.

While many studies have been small and not conducted with the highest rigor, the overall evidence to date supports the use of meditation for a variety of medical conditions.

Emotional health

Research shows that meditation can help you:

- View stressful situations differently
- Build skills that can help you manage stress
- Increase your self-awareness
- Focus on the present moment
- Reduce negative emotions

Anxiety disorders

Researchers have found that mindfulness meditation programs can help reduce anxiety.

Asthma

Mindfulness-based stress reduction (MBSR), a form of meditation and yoga, has been shown to help people manage persistent asthma when it's combined with asthma treatment. Researchers found that MBSR improved quality of life as much as treatment with widely prescribed asthma medications did.

Cancer

Research shows that people with cancer who practice MBSR are better able to cope with cancer-related stress. Although more study is needed, researchers say that MBSR is easy to learn and well-accepted by people receiving cancer treatment.

Depression

A 2014 research review involving more than 3,500 people showed that mindfulness meditation can help improve anxiety and depression.

Heart disease

Meditation has been shown to have helpful effects on the cardiovascular system because it helps reduce stress, a risk factor for heart disease. All types of meditation have been linked to a number of heart-healthy factors, including good blood pressure, blood sugar and cholesterol control.

The state of contemplation, concentration and reflection in meditation has been shown to help reduce these well-known psychological risk factors for heart disease:

- Anxiety
- Depression
- Hostility

High blood pressure

Although more study is needed, current research shows that transcendental meditation may help prevent increases in blood pressure that often happen with age.

Irritable bowel syndrome

Although the amount of improvement was small, pain and quality of life improved in people with irritable bowel syndrome as a result of mindfulness training, according to a 2013 review.

Pain

Studies are mixed on how well meditation can help reduce pain. Here's a sampling of how they differ:

- A small 2016 study showed that mindfulness meditation helps control pain when it's combined with pain medications and other approaches to pain management.
- Another 2016 study found that MBSR was more effective than typical care for low back pain.
- A review of 41 trials found that mindfulness meditation programs have potential for helping reduce pain.

Sleep problems

In a small study, adults with chronic insomnia learned MBSR and a form of MBSR designed specifically for insomnia. Sleep problems were reduced for people who practiced either type of meditation, but the MBSR designed for insomnia was shown to be more helpful than the standard MBSR. In another study, the standard form of MBSR helped people with cancer sleep better.

How to meditate: A step-by-step guide

Breath awareness is one of many tools used for meditation. Breathing is an activity that's within your control and essential to your life. That makes focusing on your breathing a convenient way to focus your attention during meditation. Use these instructions to guide your meditation practice.

1. Sit in a comfortable, dimly lit, quiet and safe place with your eyes closed.

2. Let your arms rest loosely at your side. Allow yourself a few moments to relax.

3. Pay attention to all the sounds you hear in the environment. Allow your awareness to travel to the source of the sounds. Try to avoid making any judgments about them.

4. At this point, gradually focus your attention on your breath.

5. Practice deep, slow, diaphragmatic breathing for the rest of the exercise. Breathe at a rate and depth that feels comfortable. Inhale slowly and deeply through your nose. Let the air you breathe in push your stomach out.

6. Breathe in as you slowly count to four.

7. Breathe out slowly through your mouth as you count up to six.

8. Visualize your breath at the tip of the nostril. Feel the subtle, cool breath as it flows in and a warm, cozy breath as you breathe out.

9. Keep your attention at the tip of the nostril for the next few minutes, watching the inward- and outward-flowing breath.

10. Take time to notice your breathing, gradually slowing down the rate of inhaling and exhaling as you become more comfortable.

11. Now allow your breath to become increasingly subtle until you almost stop feeling the flow.

12. Keep your awareness on the tip of the nostril with this subtle breath for the next few minutes.

13. If your thoughts start to wander, gently move your attention back to your breath.

14. Breathe out.

15. As you exhale, silently repeat to yourself:

   My breathing is smooth and rhythmic.
   My breathing is smooth and rhythmic.
   My breathing is easy and calm.
   My breathing is easy and calm.
   It feels very pleasant.

16. If you'd like, you may close your eyes and focus on each breath you take and each breath you exhale.

17. Continue to repeat to yourself:

   My breathing is smooth and rhythmic.
   My breathing is smooth and rhythmic.
   I am peaceful and calm.
   I am peaceful and calm.

Remember, if stray thoughts enter your mind, gently return your attention to the relaxation. Continue to take deep, rhythmic breaths. Let the tension fade away each time you breathe out.

Continue this exercise for as long as you like, at least 10 minutes. Throughout the exercise, remember that if stray thoughts enter your mind, gently return your attention to relaxation. Once you are ready, return to your day peaceful, more focused and relaxed.

Guided imagery

Guided imagery is a mind-body intervention that uses the power of imagination to bring about change in your physical, emotional and spiritual wellness.

With this method of meditation, you form mental images of places or situations you find relaxing. You try to use as many senses as possible, such as smells, sights, sounds and textures.

How it works

Guided imagery uses the power of your imagination to guide the way your mind and body talk to each other. By imagining certain scenes in your mind, your mind can send messages to your brain that help change the way your body feels.

The message sent to your brain is passed along to the body's endocrine, immune and autonomic nervous systems. These systems influence a wide range of bodily functions, including heart and breathing rates and blood pressure.

Using *positron emission tomography*, also known as a *PET scan*, researchers have found that the same parts of the brain are activated when people are imagining something as when they are actually experiencing it.

For example, when someone imagines a serene image, the optic cortex — the part of the brain that processes visual images — is activated in the same way as when the person is actually seeing the beautiful vista.

When you use guided imagery to imagine a beautiful vista or taking a relaxing kayak ride, the image and sensations you're creating with your mind don't just stay in your mind. They affect many parts of your body, including your heart rate, blood pressure and how your immune system functions.

How to do it

Listening to a CD that contains guided imagery coaching can be helpful. Another option is to work one-on-one or in a small group with someone trained in guided imagery who can lead you through an exercise. Guided imagery involves these four steps:

Step 1: Relax

To create a desirable image, clear your mind of all chatter, worries and distractions. Loosen tight-fitting clothing and find a comfortable, quiet place. Once you are quiet and comfortable, begin taking slow, deep breaths and release all random thoughts as you exhale.

Step 2: Concentrate

Focus your attention on your breathing as a way to clear your mind. If your mind wanders, acknowledge the thoughts that enter your mind and release them easily and effortlessly as you exhale. Then, refocus your attention on your breathing.

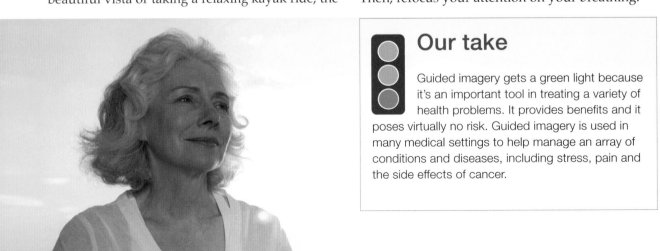

Our take

Guided imagery gets a green light because it's an important tool in treating a variety of health problems. It provides benefits and it poses virtually no risk. Guided imagery is used in many medical settings to help manage an array of conditions and diseases, including stress, pain and the side effects of cancer.

Step 3: Visualize

Now, combine a desired image with an intention, and for the next several minutes, focus on that image. You may find that your mind wanders — this may happen frequently, especially during the early stages of visualization. When it does, bring your focus back by using a slow, deep breath.

Step 4: Affirm

A positive affirmation coupled with the image will help to create a positive message that will be stored in your brain: a message you can easily recall at a later time. Combining an image with a word or phrase may help deepen your experience.

What the research says

Cancer treatment

In terms of complementary methods for treatment and prevention, cancer is an area of significant research and practice. Guided imagery is an established intervention in integrative oncology.

In one study of patients undergoing radiation therapy for breast cancer, taking part in a 30-minute guided imagery exercise led to:

- Better breathing rates
- Lower blood pressure and pulse rate

In a small study of adults managing cancer-related pain, more than half said that guided imagery helped relieve their pain. Guided imagery has been shown to reduce side effects from cancer treatment, including:

- Nausea
- Hair loss
- Depression

Stress

Guided imagery is considered an effective tool for turning on the relaxation response in people who are feeling stressed, overwhelmed or physically uncomfortable. For example, researchers recommend guided imagery as a stress management strategy to help reduce stress in people who are trying to quit smoking. Guided imagery has also been a technique that's helped reduce anxiety and offered a sense of control for people who have cancer.

Headaches

Guided imagery has been shown to be an effective and affordable way to help people who have chronic tension-type headaches. Headaches were less severe and less frequent and didn't last as long.

In terms of migraine headaches, studies have also shown that guided imagery may help reduce their frequency as effectively as taking preventive medications does.

Surgery

Research indicates that practicing guided imagery at least two to four times before surgery can reduce fear and anxiety and provide people with a greater sense of control.

In a number of studies, individuals using imagery needed less pain medication and were discharged from the hospital earlier than were those who didn't use guided imagery.

Enhancing performance

Want to improve your golf swing or piano performance? Guided imagery can help here, too. For example, in a study of 62 high school students, participants took an eight-week program that taught them cognitive skills they could use to help improve their music performance and reduce their performance anxiety. When they took time to imagine and visualize the performance, the students felt less anxious during their actual performances.

Other conditions

Guided imagery has been studied for possible use as a treatment for signs and symptoms of other medical conditions, including:

- Arthritis and other rheumatic diseases
- Heart failure
- Pregnancy

Biofeedback for stress management

Biofeedback is a technique that teaches you to control your body's functions, such as heart rate. Although it's been shown to be effective for a variety of medical conditions, biofeedback is often used as a relaxation technique. Biofeedback is used in Mayo Clinic's integrative medicine program for stress management.

With biofeedback, you're connected to electrical sensors that help you receive information about your body. This feedback helps you focus on making subtle changes in your body, such as relaxing certain muscles, to achieve the results you want, such as reducing pain.

In short, biofeedback gives you the power to use your thoughts to control your body, often to improve a health condition.

Biofeedback devices

You can receive biofeedback training in clinics and hospitals, but more and more biofeedback devices and programs are being marketed for use at home as well. Some of these are hand-held portable devices, while others connect to your computer. You can try different devices until you find one that works for you, or ask your doctor for advice. You might also check with your health insurance company to see what costs, if any, associated with biofeedback devices are covered.

Before purchasing a biofeedback device, it's important to know what these devices can — and can't — do. For example, if a manufacturer or biofeedback practitioner claims that a biofeedback device can assess your organs for disease, find impurities in your blood, cure a chronic condition or send signals into your body, check with your doctor before using it — it may not be legitimate.

Two of the main types of equipment used in biofeedback are a breathing sensor and a heart rate variability monitor. Here's how they work.

Breathing sensors

A **breathing sensor** monitors your breathing, helping you learn to breathe more slowly and

deeply. It's also been shown to reduce blood pressure.

Heart rate variability monitors

A **heart rate variability monitor** shows the increases and decreases in your heart's natural cycle or rhythm. It measures the pulse in your fingertip or earlobe and displays the time between your heartbeats. When you're stressed, the display may be jagged and spiky; when you're relaxed, the wave is smooth and consistent. By breathing more deeply and more slowly, you can change your heart rate and watch the wave change on the monitor.

For some people, biofeedback devices help produce a deep state of relaxation. Other people use biofeedback devices to assess their progress when using other practices, such as meditation.

First steps

If biofeedback is something you're interested in, talk to your doctor. Together, you can make sure that you get proper instruction and supervision and incorporate it as part of your comprehensive treatment plan. Biofeedback is personally empowering and can be a good place to start if you're not ready to sign up for a yoga class, for example. Smartphone versions of biofeedback are available that you can use anywhere.

Biofeedback appeals to people because it's usually noninvasive. It may reduce or eliminate the need for medications, and it may be a treatment alternative for people who can't tolerate medications. It also helps people take charge of their health, which may mean addressing issues of control and anxiety.

How it works

A typical biofeedback session lasts about 30 to 60 minutes. During a biofeedback session, a therapist places electrical sensors on different parts of your body. These sensors monitor your body's response to stress — for example, muscle contractions during a tension headache — and then send that information back to you through sound and visual cues.

With this feedback, you start to associate your body's response — in this case, headache pain — with certain physical sensations, such as your muscles tensing.

The next step is to learn how to invoke positive physical changes, such as relaxing muscles when your body is physically or mentally stressed. Your goal is to be able to produce these responses on your own, without a therapist or technology.

Getting started

Researchers who are looking into ways to improve heart rate variability are focusing on how biofeedback helps control your rate of breathing and improve your focus on positive emotion. They have found that biofeedback is helpful for managing stress in many ways. It can reduce the stress hormones in your body, improve symptoms of depression and post-traumatic stress disorder, improve your mood, and even enhance your job satisfaction. They're finding that biofeedback, when it's used to improve heart rate variability, can affect mental health in many ways.

If you're interested in trying biofeedback to help manage stress, HeartMath or Relaxing Rhythms are two biofeedback tools you can try on your own. When looking for a biofeedback therapist, here are some questions to ask before starting treatment:

- Are you licensed, certified or registered?
- If you aren't licensed, are you working under the supervision of a licensed health care professional?
- What is your training and experience?
- Do you have experience providing feedback for my condition?
- How many biofeedback sessions do you think I'll need?
- What's the cost, and is it covered by health insurance?
- Can you provide a list of references?

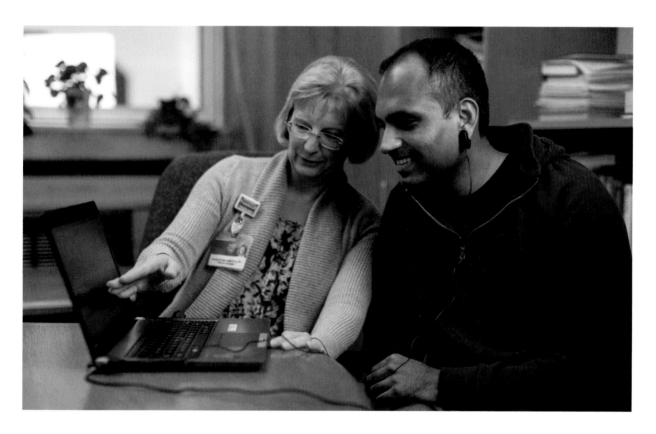

Biofeedback at Mayo Clinic

The two biofeedback techniques used most often for stress management at Mayo Clinic are:

1. **Galvanic skin response training.** Sensors measure the activity of your sweat glands and the amount of sweat on your skin, alerting you to anxiety.
2. **Heart rate variability biofeedback.** This type of biofeedback helps you control your heart rate in an effort to improve blood pressure, lung function, and stress and anxiety.

Researchers at Mayo Clinic studied the effects of biofeedback on a small group of nurses who take care of people who are critically ill.

For the study, the nurses used a biofeedback-assisted, computer-guided, self-directed meditation program for four weeks. Over those four weeks, the nurses were asked to use the meditation program four times a week for at least 30 minutes each time. Each time they used the meditation program, they were instructed to quiet their minds, observe their thoughts and cultivate positive emotions.

Nurses who took part in this program were able to improve how well they managed their stress.

Our take

Biofeedback is, for the most part, safe, widely used and accepted. It has relatively few risks, and it's practiced in many medical centers and physical therapy clinics.

Provided you receive the proper instruction and supervision, biofeedback may be useful as part of a comprehensive treatment plan.

It's important to note that some biofeedback devices may not work well if you have an underlying medical condition, such as heart rhythm problems or certain skin conditions.

What the research says

Biofeedback is useful for treating many health conditions. Studies indicate it may improve symptoms of:

- Asthma
- Raynaud's disease
- Irritable bowel syndrome
- Constipation
- Chemotherapy-related nausea and vomiting
- Incontinence
- Chronic pain
- Headache
- Anxiety
- Stress
- High blood pressure
- Stroke

Research into these and other areas is ongoing. Here's what research shows about a few applications that show the most promise.

Arthritis

People with arthritis who underwent thermal biofeedback and electromyography (EMG) biofeedback reported feeling less intense pain when their treatment was combined with cognitive behavioral therapy.

Chronic pain

Among chronic pain conditions, back pain has been the biggest focus of study. For example, some researchers have found that EMG biofeedback was more effective at treating back pain and temporomandibular disorder when compared with cognitive behavioral therapy.

Headache

Although biofeedback is helpful on its own for headaches, it's also effective when it's combined with relaxation training or cognitive behavioral therapy. Some research shows that biofeedback can be as effective as medication in preventing headaches and that it can help improve headache symptoms. Biofeedback is also helpful when combined with physical therapy.

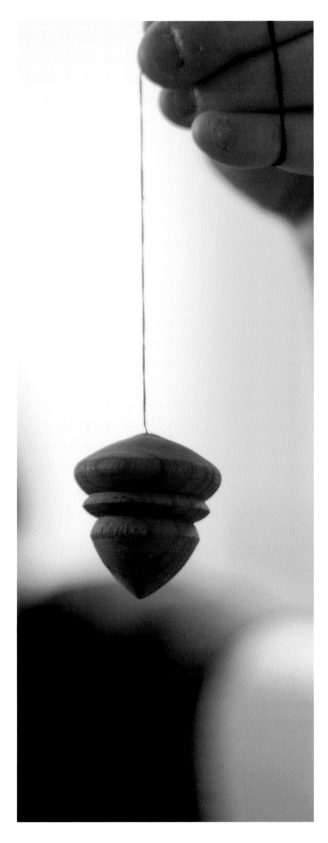

Hypnotherapy

Forms of hypnotherapy, trance and altered states of consciousness have been used by many cultures and civilizations throughout history. Today, hypnotherapy — also sometimes referred to as *hypnotic suggestion* — is seen as a trance-like state in which you have heightened focus and concentration. When you're under hypnosis, you usually feel calm and relaxed, and are more open to suggestions.

There are three stages or phases to the process of hypnotherapy:
1. Pre-suggestion
2. Suggestion
3. Post-suggestion

The goal during pre-suggestion is to open the unconscious mind to suggestion. During the second phase, a specific thought or suggestion is presented to the subject — you don't want to smoke, for example. Finally, in the post-suggestion stage, after returning to a normal state of consciousness, you practice the behavior that was suggested during hypnosis.

It's not known exactly how hypnotherapy works in the body. Changes in skin temperature, heart rate and immune response have been observed. Some scientists believe that hypnotherapy activates certain mind-body pathways in the nervous system.

While hypnotherapy is often portrayed humorously on TV and in movies, it can be an effective treatment for some people. Research shows that certain individuals connect with hypnotherapy more than others do.

Hypnotherapy can be used to help you gain control over undesired behaviors or to help you cope better with anxiety or pain. It's important to know that although you're more open to suggestion during hypnotherapy, you don't lose control over your behavior.

Are there side effects?

Hypnotherapy that's conducted by a trained therapist or health care professional is considered a safe complementary treatment. However, hypnotherapy may not be appropriate in people with severe mental illness. Adverse reactions to hypnotherapy are rare, but may include:

- Headache
- Drowsiness or dizziness
- Anxiety or distress
- Creation of false memories

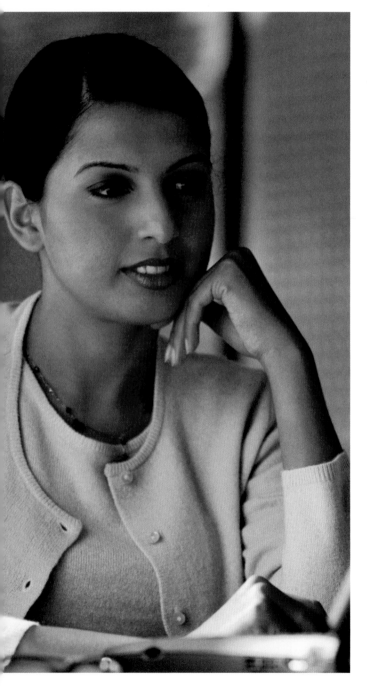

Special cautions

Use special caution before using hypnotherapy for age regression to help relive earlier events in your life. This practice remains controversial and has limited scientific evidence to support its use. It may cause strong emotions and can alter your memories or lead to creation of false memories.

In a 2015 study, Baylor University researchers found that how susceptible people are to suggestion under hypnosis plays a significant role in whether or not hypnotherapy will lead to the creation of false memories. More study needs to be done in this area, but it is a possible drawback of hypnotherapy.

Preparing for hypnotherapy

Carefully choose a therapist or health care professional to perform hypnotherapy. Get a recommendation from someone you trust. Learn as much as you can about any therapist you're considering. Start by asking questions, such as:

- Do you have training in a field such as psychology, medicine or social work?
- Are you licensed in your specialty in this state?
- How much training have you had in hypnotherapy and from what schools?
- How long have you been in practice?
- What are your fees?
- Will insurance cover your services?

You don't need any special preparation to undergo hypnotherapy, but it's a good idea to wear comfortable clothing to help you relax. Also, make sure that you're well-rested so that you're not inclined to fall asleep during the session.

How it works

During a hypnotherapy session, the following will generally take place:

Step 1

The therapist will explain the process of hypnosis and review what you hope to accomplish. Then the therapist will typically talk in a gentle, soothing tone and describe images that create a sense of relaxation, security and well-being.

Step 2

When you're in a receptive state, the therapist will suggest ways for you to achieve your goals, such as reducing pain or eliminating cravings to smoke. The therapist may also help you visualize vivid, meaningful mental images of yourself accomplishing your goals.

Step 3

When the session is over, either you're able to bring yourself out of hypnosis or your therapist helps you end your trance-like state. In general, you remain aware during your session and remember what happens under hypnosis.

Although hypnotherapy can help with a variety of conditions, it's not a magic bullet. It's typically used as one part of a broader treatment plan rather than as a stand-alone therapy.

Like any other therapy, it can be very helpful to some people and not work with others. It seems to have the most success when you're highly motivated and your therapist is well-trained and understands your particular problem.

 ## Our take

While hypnotherapy is often portrayed humorously on TV and in films, it can be an effective treatment for some people. Research indicates that some individuals are more susceptible to hypnotism than are others. Some practitioners hold that the more open you are to being hypnotized, the more likely it is that you'll benefit from the therapy. Hypnotherapy may be a reasonable choice if you need help dealing with a chronic condition. Since it poses little risk of harmful side effects, it may be worth a try.

What the research says

Hypnotherapy may offer relief to those experiencing pain associated with a number of disorders, including cancer. It is also used in treating a number of behavioral problems. In addition, it may be used to reduce anxiety before a medical or dental procedure.

Hypnotherapy can be an effective method for coping with stress and anxiety. In particular, it can reduce stress and anxiety before a medical procedure, such as a breast biopsy. Hypnotherapy has been studied for other conditions, including:

- **Pain control.** Hypnotherapy may help relieve pain associated with cancer, irritable bowel syndrome, fibromyalgia, temporomandibular joint problems (TMJ), dental procedures and headaches.
- **Hot flashes.** Hypnotherapy may relieve symptoms of hot flashes associated with menopause.
- **Behavior change.** Hypnotherapy has been used with some success in treating insomnia, bed-wetting, smoking, obesity and phobias.

Weight loss

Hypnotherapy has also been used in weight loss. Weight-loss hypnotherapy may help you shed an extra few pounds when it's part of a weight-loss plan that includes diet, exercise and counseling. But it's hard to say definitively if it works because there isn't enough solid scientific evidence that focuses specifically on weight-loss hypnotherapy.

A few studies have evaluated weight-loss hypnotherapy. Most studies show only slight weight loss, with an average loss of about 6 pounds. But the quality of some of these studies has been questioned, making it hard to determine the true effectiveness of weight-loss hypnotherapy.

Weight loss is usually best achieved through a combination of diet and exercise. If you've tried diet and exercise but are still struggling to meet your weight-loss goal, talk to your health care team about other options or lifestyle changes that you can make. Don't rely on weight-loss hypnotherapy alone because it's unlikely to lead to significant weight loss.

Spirituality

Spirituality has many definitions, and it's not necessarily connected to a specific belief system or even to religious worship. Instead, it arises from your connection with yourself and with others, the development of your personal value system, and your search for meaning in life.

For many, spirituality takes the form of religious observance, prayer, meditation or a belief in a higher power. For others, it can be found in nature, music, art or a secular community. And some people view spirituality as experiencing a sense of peace, purpose, or connection to others or nature.

No matter how you experience it, spirituality can help you find a sense of purpose and meaning within yourself and in your relationships with others. It can offer hope and peace during times of struggle or personal crisis. It can help lead to positive changes and improve your quality of life.

Spirituality and health

Spirituality and health is a growing field of study in medical education. This field of study is focused on the principles of service, compassion, dignity and interconnectedness. Aiding patients' search for meaning has become a focus in medical education and patient care, with an increasing number of spirituality and health courses, as well as research in this field.

Are you spiritual?

You probably practice spirituality every day without even realizing it. Ask yourself these questions:

- Have you connected with others, such as friends, family or a group that gathers for a spiritual purpose?
- Do you look for and do things that give your life meaning and purpose, such as the work you do or something that helps you feel connected to something larger than yourself?
- Have you helped someone in need, expecting nothing in return?
- Have you been able to see the bigger picture in life, especially during times of stress?
- Do you enjoy spending time in nature?
- Have you experienced God or a higher power at work in your life?

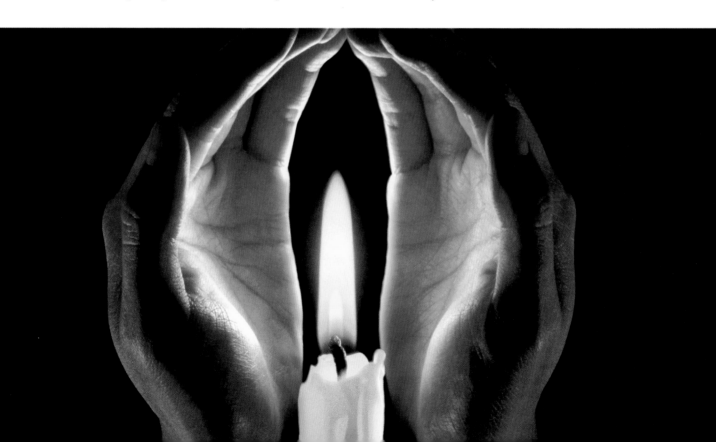

- Do you take part in activities such as prayer, meditation, deep breathing, expressing gratitude, silent observation or experiencing art?

You may be surprised to know that each and every one of these activities can be seen as a spiritual activity.

How can spirituality help with stress relief?

Spirituality can help you manage your stress and benefit your overall mental health in many ways. Here are several examples.

Sense of purpose
Spirituality can help give you a sense of purpose. Cultivating your spirituality may help uncover what's most meaningful in your life. By clarifying what's most important, you can focus less on the unimportant things and eliminate stress.

Connection to the world
Spirituality can help you connect to the world. The more you feel you have a connection in the world, the less solitary you feel — even when you're alone. This can lead to a valuable inner peace during difficult times.

Release of control
Spirituality helps you release control. When you feel part of a greater whole, you realize that you aren't responsible for everything that happens in life. You can share the burden of tough times as well as the joys of life's blessings with those around you.

Social support
Spirituality can also help you expand your support network. Whether you find spirituality in a church, mosque or synagogue, in your family, or in nature walks with a friend, this sharing of spiritual expression can help build relationships.

Healthy lifestyle
And finally, spirituality can help you lead a healthier life. People who consider themselves spiritual appear to be better able to cope with stress and heal from illness or addiction faster.

Discover your spirituality

Uncovering your spirituality may take some self-discovery. Here are some questions to ask yourself to discover what experiences and values define you.
- What are your important relationships?
- What do you value most in your life?
- What people give you a sense of community?
- What inspires you and gives you hope?
- What brings you joy?
- What are your proudest achievements?

The answers to questions such as these can help you identify the most important people and experiences in your life. Once you know the answers to these questions, you can focus your search for spirituality on the relationships and activities in life that have helped define you as a person and those that continue to inspire your personal growth.

That connection — to ourselves and to others — is how spirituality begins, and how it ultimately leads to finding a sense of purpose in life.

How to become more spiritual

Mayo Clinic has a meditation room that offers a quiet, peaceful environment for staff, patients and family members to rest, replenish and rejuvenate. With soft lighting, gentle music and the soothing sound of a water fountain, the meditation room

Our take

We are complex beings with mind, body and spirit intertwined. For many of us, our busy lives mean that spirituality sometimes gets neglected until we're confronted by a major illness. But it doesn't matter so much what brings us back to our spirituality. It's just important that we nurture all aspects of our being in our quest to stay healthy. Find ways to energize your spirit, as well as your mind and body. Doing so can bring a healthy balance to your life.

provides a transition to tranquility and contemplation. The meditation room offers the opportunity to take a moment to sit quietly and center yourself, meditate, offer prayers, talk to a friend or spiritual adviser, or write in a journal, among other spiritual opportunities.

These activities are great ways to get in touch with your own spirituality. But you don't need to be at Mayo Clinic to take steps toward becoming more spiritual. Explore your spirituality on your own with these ideas:

- Practice prayer, meditation and relaxation techniques to help you focus your thoughts.
- Keep a journal to help you express your feelings and record your progress.
- Seek out a trusted adviser or friend — someone with similar life experiences — who can help you discover what's important in life.
- Read inspirational stories or essays to help you evaluate different philosophies in life.
- Expand your horizons with new experiences in the arts if your spirituality is more secular.

What the research says

In North America, as many as 43 percent of people use prayer to improve their health.

Several hundred studies have been conducted using spirituality and prayer, and they've produced mixed results. That's because it's sometimes difficult for researchers to define various spiritual practices because they have different meaning for different people.

With that said, researchers have been able to tie spirituality to certain aspects of health and wellness. Studies show that spiritual practices may:

- Help improve range of motion and pain in people with neck pain and restricted neck movement
- Decrease feelings of hopelessness in people who have idiopathic chronic pain syndrome — a disorder defined as pain that's not related to any known disease or injury and is experienced at least once a week for three months or more
- Improve general function and reduce anxiety, depression and symptoms of many chronic health conditions

Expert insight
What is spirituality?

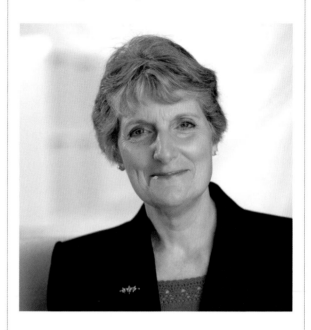

Katherine M. Piderman, Ph.D.

Mayo Clinic Hospice chaplain and coordinator of research for Chaplain Services at Mayo Clinic

Spirituality is an opportunity to experience life at the deepest level. In its best sense, spirituality offers beliefs, practices and relationships that form the way you relate to yourself and others. It gives you a way to approach each day with wonder and gratitude, grace and generosity, meaning and purpose. Spirituality helps you see the blessings in each day and helps motivate you to add to the goodness of all.

Spirituality doesn't ask you to pretend you're not suffering or in doubt. Instead, it can steady you, guide you and give you hope, even in the midst of it. In times of deep struggle, spirituality can give you the courage to pray more honestly, to meditate more deeply, or to talk with a chaplain or spiritual guide about your experience. It can also show you that it's OK to just trust in the goodness and love that's present within you.

Positive thinking

Research shows that people who have a positive outlook on life do better in the long run than do those who see things negatively. In fact, Mayo Clinic research shows that optimists even live longer than do pessimists.

On the surface, you might think that this is simply due to their underlying health — it's not hard to believe that people who are healthy might just naturally feel happier. But studies suggest that the situation works the other way around, too: Changing your attitude can have direct effects on your health.

Benefits of positive thinking

By seeing life in a positive light, you may:

- Be less likely to be depressed
- Have lower levels of distress
- Be less likely to get the common cold
- Have better psychological and physical well-being
- Have a lower risk of dying from heart disease
- Be better able to cope with hardships and stress

What makes positive thinking helpful?

Researchers don't have completely clear answers regarding why people who have a positive outlook on life experience these health benefits. One theory is that a positive attitude enables you to cope better with stressful situations, which reduces the harmful health effects of stress on your body. It's also thought that positive and optimistic people tend to live healthier lifestyles — they get more physical activity, follow a healthier diet, and don't smoke or drink alcohol in excess.

And if you think back to some of the negative effects of stress you've learned about in this book, it's not too hard to see why having a positive outlook on life can have the opposite effect of stress — and can lead to better health.

Step 1: Self-talk

Like stress, negative self-talk can have negative effects on your health. But adopting positive thinking is a habit you can adopt with practice. This may mean putting a stop to the negative messages you mentally tell yourself.

If a negative thought creeps into your mind, redirect your thoughts to something you can do right away, such as taking a short walk around the block or even taking three deep breaths.

From there, surround yourself with positive people who will help provide encouragement rather than undermine you or make you doubt yourself and your ability to achieve your goals.

One final word of advice

It may take a bit of practice to get into the habit of more positive self-talk. One simple rule is this: Don't say anything to yourself that you wouldn't say to anyone else.

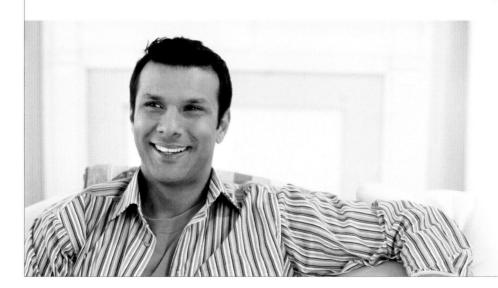

Chiropractic or osteopathic manipulation

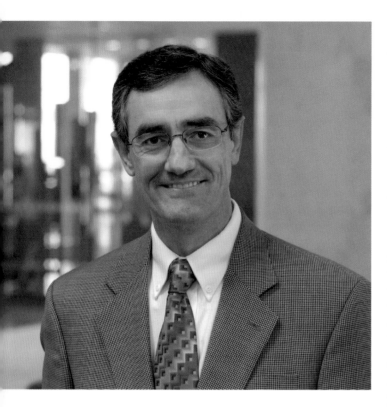

Ralph E. Gay, M.D.
Physical Medicine and Rehabilitation

Dr. Gay serves as vice chair of the Midwest Spine Care Practice in Mayo Clinic's Department of Physical Medicine and Rehabilitation in Rochester, Minnesota.

A visit with Dr. Gay

Hands-on therapies have been used to relieve pain for centuries. Of them, spinal manipulation and chiropractic care are used most often to treat musculoskeletal conditions such as back pain, neck pain and headache, although some people use it for other conditions as well.

In most countries, chiropractic care is used alongside — rather than as a replacement to — conventional medicine. This attitude is catching on more and more in the United States. The idea is that chiropractic practitioners can offer something unique from their conventional medicine counterparts. There's a clear role for chiropractors who are interested in partnering with conventional medical practitioners to offer guidance and treatment regarding musculoskeletal issues.

The field of spinal manipulation is growing in part because the evidence supporting the use of hands-on therapies is substantial. Spinal manipulation and chiropractic care have a significant body of scientific evidence supporting their use for certain conditions, such as low back pain.

Although not without risk, most hands-on treatments have limited potential for harm. When used appropriately, the most common side effect is local discomfort, which is generally short-lived. More-serious complications can happen, though. Probably the most controversial treatment is neck (cervical spine) manipulation, which in rare instances can cause stroke. Estimates suggest that this can occur from 1 in 400,000 cervical spine manipulations to 3 to 6 per 10 million cervical spine manipulations. Fortunately, providers who use spinal manipulation are some of the most highly educated complementary therapy practitioners.

Overall, spinal manipulation is a relatively safe option that has shown — and continues to show — benefits for musculoskeletal conditions. It's also reasonable in terms of cost; taken together, these benefits of chiropractic care are making this practice more accessible for those who are interested in considering it.

Chiropractic or osteopathic manipulation

Spinal manipulation, also known as *chiropractic adjustment* or *osteopathic manipulative treatment*, is practiced by chiropractors, doctors of osteopathic medicine and some physical therapists. The term *chiropractic* combines the Greek words *cheir* (meaning hand) and *praxis* (which means practice) to describe a treatment that's done by hand.

Chiropractic care is based on the idea that your body's structure — nerves, bones, joints and muscles — and its capacity for healthy function are closely intertwined. By aligning and balancing your body's structure, chiropractic treatment is intended to support the body's natural ability to heal itself. The chiropractic manipulative treatment, often called an adjustment, is intended to improve spinal mobility. The goal is to restore spinal movement and, as a result, improve function and decrease back pain.

According to the 2012 National Health Interview Survey, Americans spent $4 billion out of their own pockets on visits to practitioners of chiropractic or osteopathic manipulation. According to the American Chiropractic Association, people often go to chiropractors for neuromusculoskeletal issues, such as headaches, joint pain, neck pain, low back pain and sciatica. Chiropractors also treat patients with osteoarthritis, carpal tunnel syndrome, tendinitis, sprains and strains, although research showing conclusive benefit is lacking for many of these.

How it works

During an adjustment, chiropractors use their hands to apply a controlled force to a joint. This often results in a cracking sound made by separation of the joint surfaces. Although this sound is common, it doesn't have to occur for the treatment to be successful.

In addition, chiropractors may use muscle pressure and stretching to relax muscles that are shortened or in spasm. Many chiropractors also use treatments such as exercise, ultrasound and electrical muscle stimulation. Some chiropractors use instruments to adjust the spine, but these methods haven't been carefully studied, so their value is uncertain.

Tissue injury may be caused by a single traumatic event, such as improper lifting of a heavy object, or through repetitive stresses, such as sitting in an awkward position with poor spinal posture for an extended period of time. In either case, injury leads to physical and chemical changes that can cause inflammation, pain and loss of function. Manipulating or adjusting the affected joints and tissues can help you move those joints more easily and can help relieve pain and muscle tightness while your tissues heal.

Chiropractic care can also be used as a complement, or supporting, treatment for other medical conditions by relieving the musculoskeletal aspects associated with the condition.

History of spinal manipulation

Chiropractic care can be traced back to the beginning of recorded time. Writings from China and Greece from 2700 B.C. and 1500 B.C., respectively, mention how maneuvering the lower extremities helped ease low back pain. The Greek physician Hippocrates also wrote about the importance of spinal manipulation.

However, the practice of spinal manipulation didn't start catching on until the late 19th century. In 1895, Daniel David Palmer founded the chiropractic profession in Davenport, Iowa. Palmer was well-read in the medical journals of his time and had a lot of knowledge about developments in anatomy and physiology that were occurring throughout the world back then. He founded the Palmer School of Chiropractic in 1897.

To receive a Doctor of Chiropractic (DC) degree, a person has to complete four to five years at an accredited chiropractic college. Chiropractors also have to pass a national board exam and state board examinations before receiving a license to practice.

Safety

Chiropractic adjustment is generally considered to be safe. It occasionally causes discomfort but is safe when it's performed by someone who's trained and licensed to deliver chiropractic care. You may have mild soreness or aching following treatment, just as you would with some forms of exercise. But this soreness usually resolves within 12 to 48 hours after treatment. Some people experience minor side effects for a few days after chiropractic adjustment. These side effects may include headache, fatigue or pain in the parts of the body that were treated.

Serious complications associated with chiropractic adjustment are rare but may include a herniated disk or compression of the nerves in your lower spinal column (known as cauda equina syndrome), which can cause pain, weakness, loss of feeling in your legs or genital area, and loss of bowel or bladder control. In very rare instances, neck manipulation may cause a type of stroke known as vertebral artery dissection.

Chiropractic care is not appropriate for everyone. Don't seek chiropractic adjustment if you have severe osteoporosis, numbness, tingling or loss of strength in an arm or leg, cancer in your spine, or an increased risk of stroke.

During the adjustment

At your first visit, your chiropractor will ask questions about your health history and perform a physical exam, paying special attention to your spine. Your chiropractor may also recommend other examinations or tests, such as X-rays or laboratory tests.

During a typical chiropractic adjustment, your chiropractor will place you in specific positions to treat the affected area. You'll often lie facedown on a specially designed, padded table. The chiropractor may use his or her hands to apply a controlled force to a joint, pushing it beyond its usual range of motion. You may hear popping or cracking sounds as your chiropractor moves your joints during the treatment session.

Your chiropractor may also recommend other types of treatment, such as heat or ice, massage, stretching, electrical stimulation, exercise, or weight loss.

Although some people experience minor side effects after adjustment, spinal manipulation is generally a safe therapy — although it is not effective for everybody.

If your symptoms don't begin to improve after several weeks of treatments, chiropractic adjustment might not be the best option for you.

Our take

From a philosophical perspective, chiropractors generally belong to one of two groups: those who believe that spinal adjustment can treat most, if not all, conditions; and those who use chiropractic adjustments to treat joint and muscle problems. The scientific evidence clearly supports chiropractic treatment for musculoskeletal conditions, particularly for neck and back pain. You might consider chiropractors as musculoskeletal pain specialists.

The green light in spinal manipulation refers to use of this therapy for musculoskeletal conditions because there's no evidence to support the belief that spinal manipulation can cure whatever ails you. Select a practitioner who's willing to work with other members of your health care team.

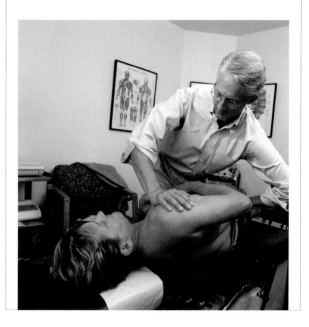

What the research says

Numerous well-designed studies have shown that spinal manipulation is an effective treatment for mild to moderate low back pain. Spinal manipulation is also used to treat other conditions. There's some evidence it may improve headache symptoms or help relieve neck pain. As for treatment of nonmusculo-skeletal conditions, such as asthma or ear infections, studies either haven't been conducted or haven't found spinal manipulation to be effective.

Back pain

Many randomized studies have been conducted to examine the effect of spinal manipulation on back pain. Most studies have found that it does help. In a recent systematic review, researchers studied 26 randomized controlled trials that included more than 6,000 participants to determine what effect spinal manipulation has on chronic low back pain. In this review, researchers found that spinal manipulation is as effective as other common back pain therapies, such as exercise and standard medical care.

Other conditions

In 2010, researchers reviewed scientific evidence on manual therapies for a range of conditions. They found that spinal manipulation and mobilization may help treat several conditions in addition to back pain. Migraines and neck-related headaches, neck pain, upper- and lower-extremity joint conditions, and whiplash-associated disorders all made the list.

What doesn't spinal manipulation help?

The 2010 research review also identified a number of conditions that spinal manipulation or mobilization doesn't seem to help. These conditions included asthma, high blood pressure and menstrual pain. For a number of symptoms and conditions, including fibromyalgia, midback pain, sciatica and temporo-mandibular joint disorder (TMJ), researchers couldn't say if treatment was helpful or not.

Safety

Researchers are continuing to study the safety of chiropractic treatment. A 2007 study of almost 20,000 people who received chiropractic treatment in the United Kingdom showed that minor side effects after cervical spine manipulation — such as temporary soreness — were relatively common, but that the risk of a serious adverse event was low or very low up to seven days after treatment.

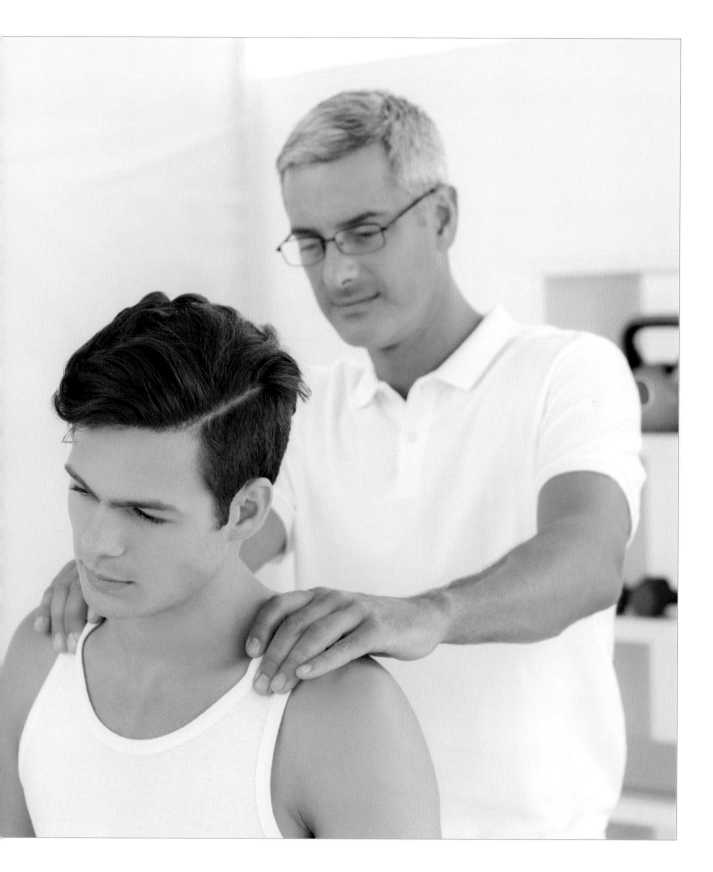

Massage therapy

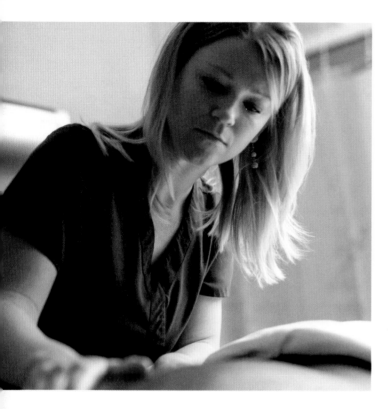

Jennifer L. Hauschulz, BCTMB
Integrative Medicine and Health

Jennifer is one of several massage therapists who offer massage therapy in both inpatient and outpatient settings in Rochester, Minnesota.

A visit with Jennifer Hauschulz

Massage is a bodywork technique that is well-known for its benefits in relieving pain and stress. But it's also used for a number of other conditions, including digestive disorders and fibromyalgia, as well as after surgery and alongside cancer treatment.

As researchers learn more about its benefits, massage therapy is being offered more and more in hospitals and has even been shown to help improve blood glucose levels in people with diabetes, as well as improve lung function in children who have asthma.

Just as it's critical to find the right fit when you're choosing a doctor or another medical specialist, choosing a massage therapist who will fit your needs is an important part of the process when you're considering massage therapy.

Although not all massage therapists are required to be board certified, you can find a list of board-certified massage therapists in your area by visiting the National Certification Board for Therapeutic Massage & Bodywork's website (*www.ncbtmb.org*). If you're interested in finding a massage therapist who has experience in working with people who have cancer, the Society for Oncology Massage (*http://s4om.org*) is a helpful resource. From there, look for a massage therapist who will talk with you thoroughly and tailor your massage to your specific situation.

Although there have been many exciting developments in the field of massage therapy, in this section you'll also learn about other techniques — some of which are often directly used in massage, such as aromatherapy, as well as related techniques.

In this section, you'll learn that many different types of bodywork techniques may aid in your overall wellness.

Massage therapy

Massage has been used for thousands of years in many cultures to heal, soothe and relieve pain. Combined, massage therapy providers represent the largest group of organized complementary care practitioners in the United States and Canada.

Massage is a general term for pressing, rubbing and manipulating your skin, muscles, tendons and ligaments. Massage therapists typically use their hands and fingers for massage, but may also use their forearms, elbows and even feet. Massage may range from light stroking to deep pressure.

Today, massage is being offered more frequently along with standard treatment for a wide range of medical conditions and situations. A massage may make you feel relaxed, and most people use it for relaxation. But it isn't likely to cure everything that ails you. And if performed incorrectly, it could hurt you. Learning about massage before you try one can help ensure that the experience is safe and enjoyable (see "What to expect during a massage" on the next page).

Common types of massage

There are many different types of massage. Here are four of the most common:

1. **Swedish massage** is the most popular kind of massage. It's a gentle form of massage that uses long strokes, kneading, deep circular movements, vibration and tapping to help you feel relaxed and energized.
2. **Deep massage** is a technique that uses slower, more-forceful strokes to target the deeper layers of muscle and connective tissue. It's commonly used to help with muscle damage from injuries.
3. **Sports massage** is like Swedish massage, but it's geared toward preventing or treating injuries for people involved in sports activities.
4. And finally, **trigger point massage** focuses on tight muscle fibers that can form if you've injured or overused a muscle.

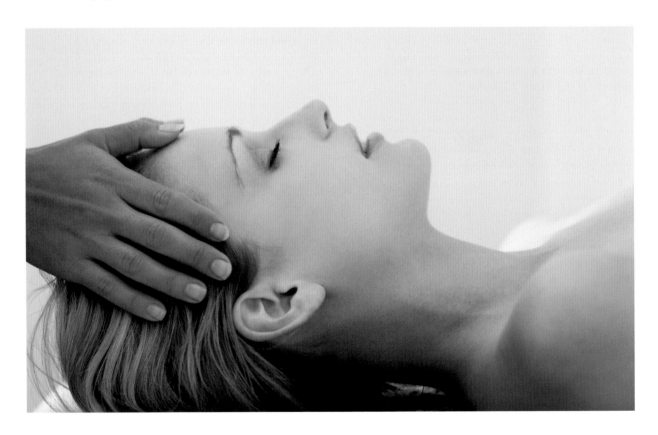

What to expect during a massage

At a massage therapy session, here's what you're likely to expect:

- **You'll likely need to answer a few questions.** Your massage therapist will want to know what you hope to gain from your massage. For example, are you looking for help with a pulled muscle? Your massage therapist will also want to know about any medical conditions you might have.
- **You may need to undress or wear loosefitting clothing.** Undress only to the point that you're comfortable. You generally lie on a table and cover yourself with a sheet.
- **Most of the time, you will lie on your stomach at the beginning of your massage and then flip over halfway through.** The therapist may use pillows or bolsters to take strain off your lower back and allow you to relax completely during the massage.
- **Depending on preference, your massage therapist may use oil or lotion to reduce friction on your skin.** Tell your massage therapist if you might be allergic to any ingredients or are sensitive to certain scents.
- **You can also have a massage while sitting in a chair that's specially made to slope forward so the therapist can work on your back while you're fully clothed.** Your massage therapist should perform an evaluation through touch to locate painful or tense areas and to determine how much pressure to apply.
- **Your massage session may last anywhere from 15 to 90 minutes, depending on the type of massage and how much time you have.** No matter what kind of massage you choose, you should feel calm and relaxed during and after your massage.
- **Finally, keep in mind that you shouldn't feel significant pain during a massage.** If a massage therapist is pushing too hard, ask for lighter pressure. Occasionally, you may have a sensitive spot in a muscle that feels like a knot. It's likely to be uncomfortable while your massage therapist works it out. But if it becomes painful, speak up.

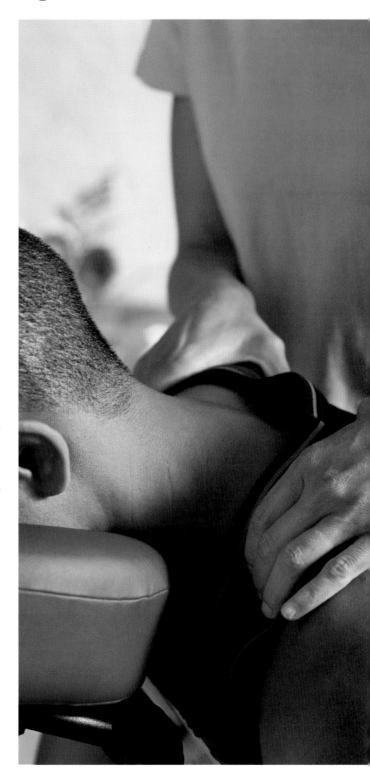

Massage at Mayo Clinic

Massage therapy is one of several integrative medicine treatments used in Mayo Clinic's Integrative Medicine and Health Program to promote physical, mental and spiritual wellness.

How is massage used?

Trained specialists at Mayo Clinic offer massage therapy for a variety of conditions. Massage can:

- Decrease swelling and impaired joint mobility
- Ease muscle spasms and muscle tension
- Increase circulation to promote healing
- Reduce pain and improve muscle tone

In addition, many of Mayo Clinic's massage therapists have been trained in:

- Acupressure (see page 142)
- Reflexology (see page 143)
- Mobilization of scar tissue
- Oncology massage
- Lymphatic drainage (or lymphatic massage)

Doctors and massage therapists at Mayo Clinic work together to coordinate a massage therapy treatment plan for an injury or a condition as part of an individual's overall plan of care. Massage therapy is used for:

- Stress
- Anxiety
- Pain
- Low back pain
- Fibromyalgia
- Soft tissue strains or injuries
- Upper back and neck tightness or pain
- Temporomandibular joint (TMJ) pain
- Digestive disorders
- Stress-related insomnia
- Headaches
- Paresthesia and nerve pain
- Myofascial pain syndrome
- Sports injuries

Mayo Clinic research on massage therapy

Mayo Clinic researchers have conducted several studies to discover the most effective uses of massage therapy. Two studies measured the effect of massage therapy on reducing pain, anxiety and tension in people undergoing heart surgery. In another study, led by a Mayo Clinic massage therapist, massage therapy was offered to people undergoing chest surgery.

These studies showed that massage helped reduce pain and decrease anxiety. This research led surgeons to make massage therapy a routine part of care following open-heart surgery.

In another study, a massage therapist interviewed 160 patients and was able to apply massage therapy to each patient in a way that suited each person's individual needs. The people who received massage therapy for this study reported having dramatically lower levels of pain and were easier to care for. Mayo Clinic researchers also studied the effects of a 20-minute massage on patients preparing to have a cardiac catheterization, a procedure that's often stressful for those receiving it. In fact, just the thought of this procedure can make people nervous. In this type of situation, feeling as calm and relaxed as possible is best for everyone — patients, doctors and nurses alike. In this study of 130 patients, researchers found that patients who received a 20-minute massage just 30 minutes before the procedure had less pain, were less anxious and tense, and were more satisfied with their experience overall.

From there, similar studies were conducted for other types of surgery. Ultimately, the Mayo Clinic Department of Surgery added more massage therapists to make massage therapy part of its standard of care. Today, all Mayo Clinic patients can request massage therapy as part of their hospital care.

Massage therapy for all

Massage therapy at Mayo Clinic isn't limited to patients. Working in a hospital is stressful for nurses, so Mayo Clinic launched a pilot trial, offering chair massage for nurses working in the fibromyalgia and inpatient psychiatric units. For this trial, nurses were given a 15-minute chair massage.

Researchers discovered a dramatic decrease in stress-related symptoms and anxiety, and almost 80 percent of the nurses said they felt that their overall job satisfaction improved because of massages.

What makes massage effective?

Massage is an effective treatment for several different reasons. First, muscles and tissues are being manipulated in a structured and purposeful way. Moving muscles and the fibers that connect them can help reduce pain or assist in aligning the body or improving posture. Second, massage harnesses the power of human touch, a key benefit of massage therapy.

Environment

The massage therapy environment may also play a role in the healing power of massage. For instance:

- Massage usually occurs in a very quiet, pleasant environment.
- Sometimes aromatherapy also is used, evoking certain healing sensations (see page 90).
- Pleasant and relaxing music often is playing during a massage therapy session.
- Natural treatments and plants also may be present, helping to promote thoughts of health and healing.

Effects on well-being

In most studies of massage therapy, researchers have found that people say their overall well-being is improved. A number of studies also suggest that massage makes positive changes to the body, including a decrease in some of the chemicals associated with stress, such as cortisol.

Beyond its specific treatment benefits, massage is something that people enjoy because it often involves caring, comfort, a sense of empowerment, and creating deep connections with a massage therapist.

Despite the many benefits of massage, this therapy isn't meant as a replacement for conventional medical care. As with other integrative therapies, tell your doctor you're trying massage and be sure to follow any standard treatment plans for specific medical conditions. In certain circumstances, massage therapy can pose risks, which you'll learn about on the next page.

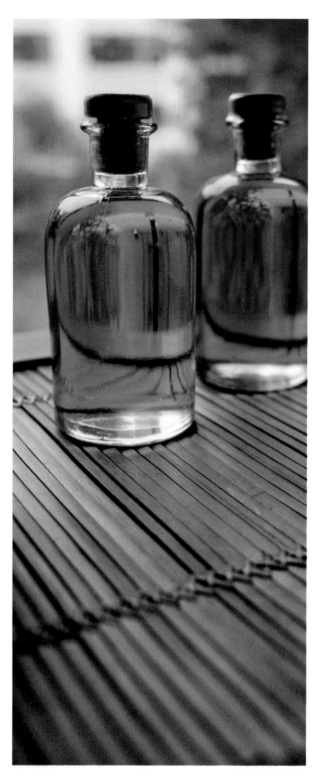

Risks of massage

Most people can benefit from massage, but it's not appropriate for everyone. If you have had a recent heart attack, have a bleeding disorder, or are taking blood-thinning medication, talk to your doctor first. Also talk to your doctor before trying massage if you have deep vein thrombosis, burns, fractures or severe osteoporosis; in these cases, massage may be harmful. Massage should not be applied directly to cancerous tumors. People with healing wounds or nerve damage should avoid pressure on affected areas of the body.

Be sure to talk about the pros and cons of massage with your doctor, especially if you are pregnant or have cancer or unexplained pain.

Some forms of massage can leave you feeling a bit sore the next day. But in general, massage shouldn't be painful or uncomfortable. If any part of your massage doesn't feel right or is painful, speak up right away. Most serious problems come from too much pressure during massage.

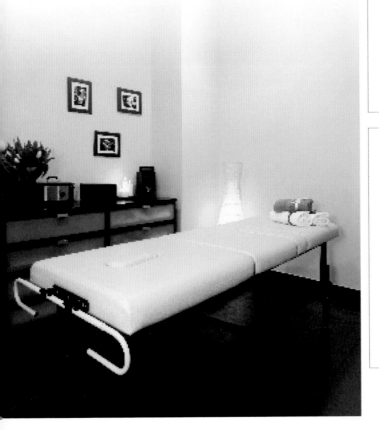

Finding a massage therapist

Several types of health care professionals — such as physical therapists, occupational therapists and massage therapists — perform massage.

Ask your doctor or someone else you trust for a recommendation. Most states regulate massage therapists through licensing, registration or certification requirements.

Don't be afraid to ask a potential massage therapist questions such as these:

- Are you licensed, certified or registered?
- What is your training and experience?
- How many massage therapy sessions do you think I'll need?
- What's the cost, and is it covered by health insurance?

Watch now

Get Dr. Bauer's take not only on the benefits of massage but also tips for finding a massage therapist in this video interview with the American Massage Therapy Association:

https://www.youtube.com/watch?v=LDkMlZX_XVc

Our take

Almost everyone feels better after a massage. Massage has been shown to help treat many conditions and boost overall wellness in a number of ways.

There are different types of massage. If you find one that works for you, you may be surprised at how quickly it can become a regular part of your wellness routine. While massage therapy is generally safe, there are some instances in which a massage may not be recommended.

What the research says

Researchers have found that massage is an effective way to reduce stress, pain and muscle tension. It releases endorphins — the body's natural painkillers — and increases the blood flow through your body. It can also reduce heart rate and improve how well your immune system works.

More research on the benefits of massage is needed, but the studies that have been done so far indicate that massage may be helpful for:

Pain
Researchers have found that massage is useful for chronic low back pain, chronic neck pain, rheumatoid arthritis, osteoarthritis of the knee, burns and pain following heart surgery. In one small study of about 60 adults with chronic low back pain, researchers found that the use of massage may potentially help reduce

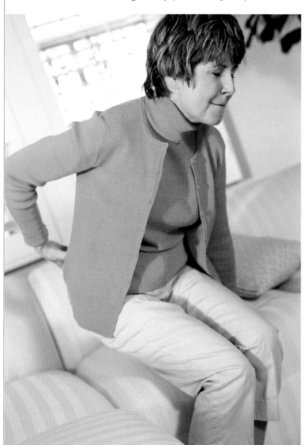

the use of anti-inflammatory medication used to treat low back pain.

Fibromyalgia
In terms of pain management, fibromyalgia has been a specific area of study for massage research. Although more study is needed, researchers see potential benefits in the use of massage to help relieve symptoms of this condition.

A 2010 review found that massage therapy may be useful for treating fibromyalgia by helping temporarily reduce pain, as well as other symptoms related to this condition, including fatigue.

Heart health
In addition to helping relieve pain following heart surgery, massage may be therapeutic from a prevention standpoint as well. Massage therapy has been shown to help lower blood pressure and manage stress, which can help promote heart health.

Mental health and wellness
Massage therapy offers benefits for a number of mental health conditions, including depression, anxiety and stress. Research also shows that massage can help people coping with seasonal affective disorder by improving mood and boosting energy levels.

Aging
Studies show that massage therapy offers benefits for people of any age. More and more aging adults look to massage therapy as a way to treat aches and pains and help manage chronic pain and long-term care. Researchers have found that regular massage can help promote relaxation and stability and even lessen the effects of dementia, high blood pressure and osteoarthritis.

Cancer
Massage therapy may reduce pain, improve mood, promote relaxation and improve sleep in people with cancer. A massage therapist must take special precautions when treating someone with cancer, but it has been shown to be therapeutic.

Aromatherapy

Aromatherapy is based on the idea that certain scents can affect your psychological or physical well-being.

Because scent is connected to memory, many people think that imagining a smell that makes you feel good is aromatherapy. While this is part of aromatherapy, other factors are involved, as well. Another side to the practice of aromatherapy is focused on the therapeutic use of essential oils extracted from plants.

How essential oils work

Essential oils are concentrated extracts taken from the roots, leaves, seeds or blossoms of plants. Each essential oil contains its own mix of active ingredients, and this mix determines what the oil is used for. Some oils are used to promote physical healing — for example, to treat swelling or fungal infections.

Other plant oils can help you relax or make a room smell pleasant. Lavender oil, for example, contains a large amount of an active ingredient that's thought to be calming. Highly concentrated oils may be inhaled directly or indirectly or applied to the skin through massage, lotions or bath salts.

Essential oils have been used for therapeutic purposes for thousands of years.

Essential oil safety

Essential oils used in aromatherapy aren't regulated by the Food and Drug Administration, but they're generally considered safe. However, just because they're natural doesn't mean that they don't pose risks if they're used inappropriately. It can be harmful to overuse or ingest essential oils, and they may produce some side effects or interactions.

Inhaling essential oils isn't likely to be toxic, but you may be sensitive to an essential oil if you're in a nonventilated room, the temperature is very high, and there is a constant diffusion of essential oil that saturates the air.

Essential oils are often applied to the skin, so it's important to know about adverse skin reactions they may cause. Essential oils can cause allergic reactions, skin irritation and sun sensitivity. It's unknown how safe or effective oils are when taken orally.

With aromatherapy massage, the idea is that your skin is able to absorb the essential oils at the same time you're breathing in their scent and while you're experiencing the physical benefits of the massage.

Common aromatherapy scents used for relaxation include lavender, jasmine, chamomile, bergamot, rose, sandalwood and vanilla.

Aromatherapy at Mayo Clinic

At Mayo Clinic, aromatherapy is used in a variety of ways. For example, a sample of lavender is offered to patients who are feeling nervous or anxious before a procedure. Inhaling the scent of lavender can help ease anxiety and enhance overall relaxation. Lavender samples may also be offered to help with sleeplessness and as a way to help manage pain. In other cases, spearmint and ginger may help manage nausea. Essential oils also may be used with other integrative medicine therapies, such as massage, acupuncture or stress management counseling.

Our take

Research on the effectiveness of aromatherapy is limited. However, when used appropriately, aromatherapy is generally safe to use. It can often bring a sense of comfort, and in some cases, it can have a direct impact on specific symptoms.

What the research says

The few formal studies of aromatherapy that have been done on humans suggest that aromatherapy may offer a number of health benefits.

Anxiety
Some studies have shown aromatherapy can help relieve anxiety.

Depression
Some studies have shown aromatherapy can help relieve symptoms of depression. When massage therapy is used in addition to medications or psychotherapy, the use of essential oils seems to help. The benefits seem to be related to relaxation caused by the scents and the massage.

Quality of life
Some studies have shown aromatherapy can improve quality of life, especially for people who have chronic health conditions.

Dialysis
Smaller studies suggest that aromatherapy with lavender oil may help make needle sticks less painful for people receiving dialysis.

Sleep
Smaller studies suggest that aromatherapy with lavender oil may improve sleep for people who are hospitalized.

Pain
Smaller studies suggest that aromatherapy with lavender oil may reduce pain for children undergoing tonsillectomy.

Pregnancy
Clinical studies involving qualified midwives showed that when the midwives used essential oils — in particular, rose, lavender and frankincense — pregnant women felt less anxiety and fear, had a stronger sense of well-being, and needed less pain medication during delivery. Some of the women also said that peppermint oil helped relieve nausea and vomiting during labor.

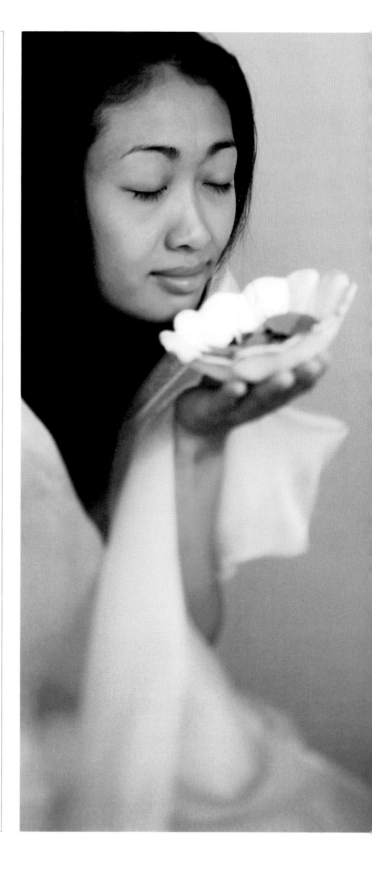

Chinese massage (Tui na)

The oldest known system of massage, tui na has been used in China for thousands of years and is closely related to acupuncture and acupressure.

The term *tui na* literally means "push and pull" in Chinese. It's a series of maneuvers that include pressing, kneading and grasping, which range from light stroking to deep tissue work. The maneuvers involve hand techniques to massage the body's soft tissues (muscles and tendons).

Tui na and other forms of massage

Tui na is unlike other forms of massage therapy but similar to acupuncture and acupressure because it uses the meridian system. Through the application of massage and manipulation techniques at specific points on the body, the goal of tui na is to re-establish the normal flow of *qi*, discussed on page 96.

Unlike most forms of massage, Chinese massage generally isn't a light, relaxing massage. It can be very powerful, and some people find parts of the massage to be a bit painful. It's generally used to treat injuries, joint and muscle problems, chronic pain, and some internal disorders. It shouldn't be used for conditions such as a bone fracture or an external wound or open sores. It's also not recommended to treat life-threatening conditions, such as a cancerous tumor.

Our take

Tui na has been part of a comprehensive traditional Chinese medicine system for thousands of years. However, limited research has focused on its effect and potential benefits.

Some small studies suggest that tui na may offer health and wellness benefits. However, more research is needed before it can become a recommended integrative therapy.

What the research says

Of the limited research that has been done on tui na, studies show that it may be effective in helping treat these conditions.

High blood pressure
When used with medication, research shows that tui na can help lower blood pressure in people who have hypertension. However, researchers in one study are cautious about these findings because of the poor quality of information available.

Low back pain
A randomized controlled trial showed that tui na, when combined with herbal ointment, can help treat low back pain more effectively than massage therapy can on its own. These researchers were also cautious about these results, echoing the need for longer-term, better-quality studies on the use of tui na for low back pain.

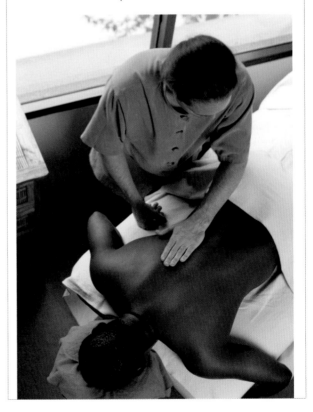

Rolfing

Rolfing, also referred to as structural integration, is a form of bodywork developed by Ida P. Rolf, Ph.D. It's based on the theory that the tissues surrounding your muscles become thickened and stiff as you get older. This affects your posture and how well you're able to move. Although it loosens tight tissues, reduces stress and offers a feeling of relaxation like massage does, the idea behind Rolfing is to align and balance the different parts of the body in a way that helps your body function smoothly in a coordinated fashion.

How Rolfing works

Rolfing practitioners use their fingers, knuckles, thumbs, elbows and knees to slowly manipulate muscles and the tissues surrounding muscles and joints in an effort to alter a person's posture and realign the body. Rolfing may relieve stress and anxiety, ease pain, improve posture and balance, or help you create more-refined patterns of movement.

People with bleeding disorders or who are taking blood thinners should avoid Rolfing. Pregnant women and those with broken bones, osteoporosis, an implanted medical device such as a shunt or a pacemaker, eczema, psoriasis, a skin infection, deep vein thrombosis, burns or open wounds, or uncontrolled mental illness, should also avoid Rolfing. If you have questions about whether Rolfing is safe for you, talk with your health care team.

Our take

Some people find Rolfing to be very helpful, improving their posture or helping them to feel more limber. But the therapy can also be painful.

If you have a specific underlying illness, such as advanced osteoporosis, the deep massage of Rolfing may also pose some risk. Therefore, it's best to talk to your doctor before trying Rolfing.

What the research says

Rolfing is used to treat many diseases and conditions. However, there is very limited research as to its effectiveness. It has been studied for the treatment of low back pain, cerebral palsy and chronic fatigue syndrome. The studies were small, and more reliable data are needed.

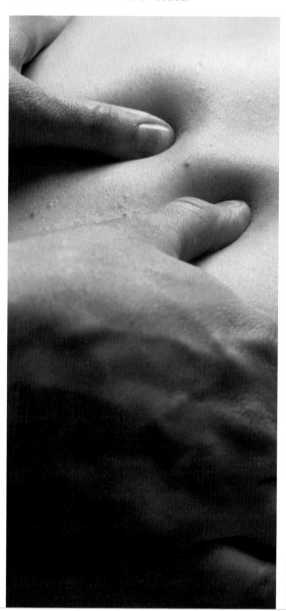

Acupuncture

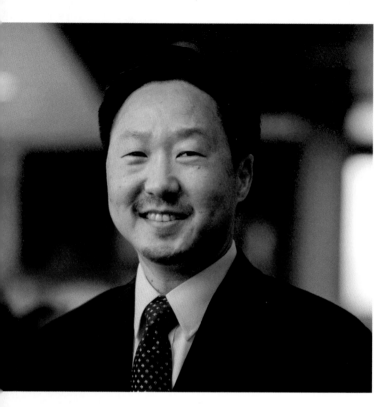

Tony Y. Chon, M.D.
General Internal Medicine

Dr. Chon is the co-medical director of Integrative Medicine and Health at Mayo Clinic in Rochester, Minnesota.

A visit with Dr. Chon

Acupuncture has been used around the world for thousands of years, but it's been only since the 1970s that it has started to become popular in the United States.

In this section, you'll discover what current research shows regarding acupuncture's effectiveness in treating a variety of ailments. First and foremost, you'll learn that the needles used for acupuncture are nothing like the needles used for other medical procedures. They're much thinner, and people often don't feel them inserted at all.

Today, acupuncture is used to treat an array of medical conditions. But in my clinical experience, acupuncture is often brought up as a last resort, long after other treatments have been tried and haven't helped.

However, a transition is taking place. More and more people are considering acupuncture as an early treatment option along with other traditional therapies for conditions where pain is a common comorbidity. Even in situations where the management of chronic pain is a struggle, acupuncture is gathering bigger momentum as a treatment option. The opioid epidemic that America is facing has highlighted the greater need for nonopioid-based therapies. In addition, people are starting to consider acupuncture for overall wellness, including stress management.

Maybe you don't have a condition you'd like to try to treat with acupuncture, but you're interested in maintaining your wellness. In addition to adopting healthy-eating habits and taking steps to manage your stress, you may consider trying integrative types of physical activity, such as yoga, tai chi or qi gong. In this type of wellness approach, acupuncture can be a good fit.

Acupuncture can be a regular practice that can produce stress-relieving effects to help you now, as well as long-term. As you'll learn in this section, acupuncture is one more way you can invest in your health and well-being.

Acupuncture

Acupuncture involves the insertion of very thin needles to various depths at strategic points on your body. According to the National Institutes of Health, at least 3 million adults nationwide receive acupuncture each year.

How it works

How acupuncture works is not entirely understood. However, current ideas about acupuncture offer some explanation.

The classical Chinese explanation starts with the idea that channels of energy run in regular patterns throughout the body and over its surface. These energy channels, or pathways, are called meridians, and they flow through your body like rivers, nourishing your body's tissues. Qi (pronounced CHEE) — defined as vital energy or life force believed to regulate your spiritual, emotional, mental and physical health — is believed to flow through these pathways and throughout your body. Because qi is thought to bring balance to various aspects of your health, an obstruction in your meridians is like a dam that backs up, causing an imbalance that leads to a blockage in the flow of qi. Acupuncture is meant to remove blockages in the flow of qi and restore and maintain health.

Many Western practitioners offer a different viewpoint on what happens in the body during acupuncture. They view the acupuncture points as places to stimulate nerves, muscles and connective tissue. Some believe that this stimulation boosts your body's natural painkillers and increases blood flow.

What happens during treatment

Most traditional Chinese medicine practitioners take a detailed history, look at your tongue, check your pulse, and come up with a full plan to restore balance. That plan will likely include acupuncture, but it is also likely to include recommendations about diet and lifestyle. And it might also include herbs, massage or exercises, such as tai chi or qi gong.

During treatment, between five and 20 needles are commonly used. You'll most likely sit or lie on a special table for 15 or 20 minutes with the needles in place. Afterwards, you might feel a little lightheaded, but you generally should also experience a sense of deep relaxation.

The number of treatments needed differs from person to person and depends on the condition being treated and how severe it is. In general, it's common to receive six to eight treatments. For complex or long-standing conditions, one or two treatments a week for several months may be recommended. For acute problems, fewer visits are usually required.

Safety

The risks of acupuncture are low if you're working with a competent, certified acupuncture practitioner. Common side effects include soreness or minor bleeding or bruising where the needles were inserted.

Acupuncture is not suitable for everyone. You may be at risk of complications if you:
- **Have a bleeding disorder.** You may experience increased risk of bleeding or bruising from the needles if you have a bleeding disorder or if you're taking blood thinners.
- **Have a pacemaker.** When acupuncture involves applying mild electrical pulses to the needles, this can interfere with a pacemaker's operation.
- **Are pregnant.** Some types of acupuncture are thought to stimulate labor, which could result in a premature delivery.

Most people feel only minimal pain as the needles are inserted; some feel no pain at all. Once the needles are in place, you generally shouldn't feel any pain. The risk of bruising and skin irritation is less than what you'd experience from a traditional hollow, hypodermic needle. Single-use, disposable needles are now the practice standard — so the risk of infection is minimal.

Preparing for acupuncture

On the day of your acupuncture treatment, there are steps you can take to help prepare yourself. This advice comes from the American Academy of Medical Acupuncture, the professional society of doctors in North America who have incorporated acupuncture into their traditional medical practice.

- Don't eat an unusually large meal right before or after your treatment.
- Don't exercise vigorously, engage in sexual activity or consume alcoholic beverages within six hours before or after treatment.
- Plan your activities so that after your treatment, you can get some rest — or at least not have to work at top performance. This is especially important for the first few visits.
- Continue to take any prescription medicines as directed by your doctor. Abusing drugs or alcohol, especially in the week before treatment, will seriously interfere with the effectiveness of acupuncture treatments.
- Remember to keep good mental or written notes of your response to treatment. This is important for your doctor to know so that the follow-up treatments can be designed to best help you.

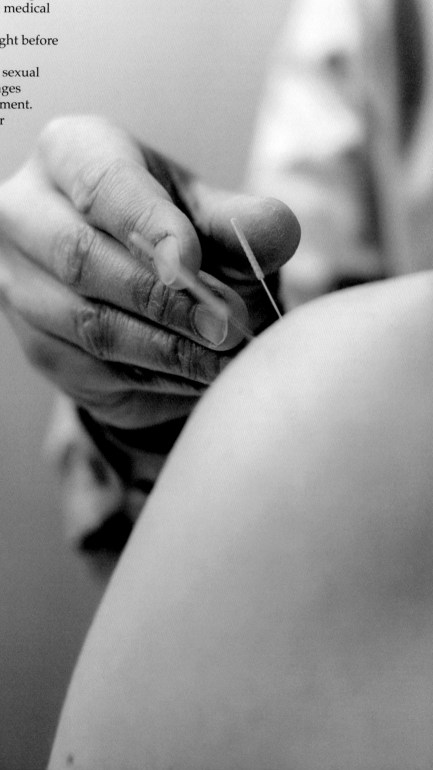

Working with a practitioner

If you're considering acupuncture, it's important to find a qualified practitioner. Take the same steps you would to take choose a doctor:

- Don't be afraid to tell your primary care doctor that you're considering acupuncture. He or she may be able to tell you about the success rate of using acupuncture for your condition or recommend a practitioner.
- Ask people you trust for recommendations.
- Check the practitioner's training and credentials. Most states require that acupuncturists who aren't physicians pass an exam conducted by the National Certification Commission for Acupuncture and Oriental Medicine.
- Interview the practitioner. Ask what's involved in the treatment, how likely it is to help your condition and how much it will cost.
- Find out whether your insurance covers the treatment.

Choosing a practitioner

Keep in mind that each person who performs acupuncture has a unique style, often blending aspects of Eastern and Western medical approaches. To help determine the type of acupuncture treatment that may help you the most, your practitioner may ask you about your symptoms, behaviors and lifestyle. An acupuncture practitioner will closely examine the parts of your body that are painful and use several very specific tools to make a diagnosis.

What happens before treatment

An acupuncture practitioner will pay attention to the color of your face. Your Western-trained physician is checking this, too — a very pale complexion may indicate anemia or shock, whereas a very ruddy one might suggest Cushing syndrome; jaundice causes a yellowish tint. An acupuncture practitioner may also carefully examine the shape, coating and color of your tongue. Another diagnostic tool is the pulse in your wrist. Traditional Chinese medicine has an elaborate system of diagnosis based on characteristics of the pulse. With this in mind, your acupuncture practitioner may examine its strength, rhythm, and quality.

An initial acupuncture evaluation may take up to 60 minutes. Subsequent appointments usually take about a half-hour.

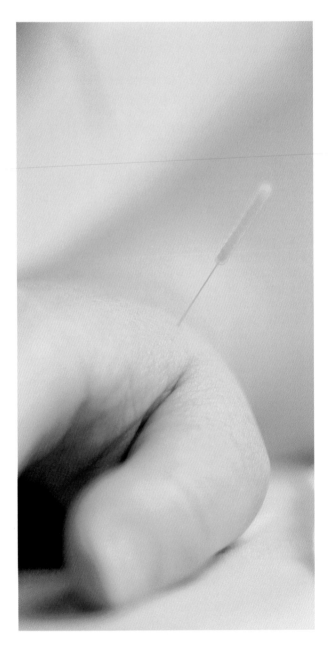

What to expect during acupuncture

Acupuncture points are situated in all areas of the body. Sometimes the appropriate points are far removed from the area of your pain.

Your acupuncture practitioner will tell you the general site of the planned treatment and whether you need to remove any clothing. A gown, towel or sheet will be provided. You'll lie on a padded table for the treatment.

You may feel a mild aching sensation when a needle reaches the correct depth. Your practitioner may gently move or twirl the needles after placement or apply heat or mild electrical pulses to the needles.

There is usually no discomfort when the needles are removed.

After an acupuncture treatment, some people feel relaxed, while others feel energized. But not everyone responds to acupuncture. If your symptoms don't begin to improve within a few weeks, acupuncture may not be right for you.

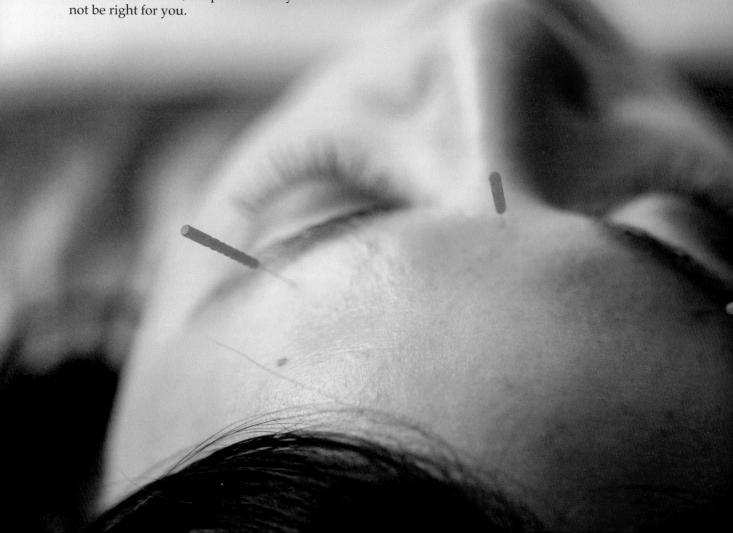

Acupuncture at Mayo Clinic

Acupuncture has been used at Mayo Clinic since the mid-1990s. Today, several licensed acupuncturists are on staff.

A number of rooms are dedicated to acupuncture at Mayo Clinic. Because a primary goal of Mayo Clinic acupuncturists is to ensure that the patient is comfortable, acupuncturists take time to talk to patients about why they were referred to acupuncture and discuss what goals a patient is hoping to accomplish through treatment. Acupuncturists at Mayo Clinic also ensure that there is no reason why acupuncture generally shouldn't be used. After all of this has taken place, the patient may or may not need to disrobe, depending on which acupuncture points need to be accessed.

Creating a relaxing environment

Mayo Clinic acupuncture practitioners try to create an optimal relaxation response while the needles are being placed. Treatment rooms have soft music and gentle lighting and, if it's preferred, a video of nature scenes can be shown during treatment.

Where is acupuncture offered?

Acupuncture is offered throughout Mayo Clinic hospitals and at Rejuvenate Spa at the Mayo Clinic Healthy Living Program at the Dan Abraham Healthy Living Center. It may be used to help treat nausea after surgery or to help with the side effects of chemotherapy.

What Mayo Clinic research shows

Acupuncture isn't just a treatment offered to patients, however. It's also a topic of interest for Mayo Clinic researchers, who have conducted several studies on how acupuncture affects patients.

In one study, researchers focused on acupuncture and fibromyalgia pain. Fibromyalgia is a disorder that involves widespread musculoskeletal pain accompanied by fatigue, sleep, memory and mood issues. Researchers believe that fibromyalgia amplifies painful sensations by affecting the way the brain processes pain signals.

The widespread pain of fibromyalgia can be difficult to treat with medication alone. However, acupuncture has been shown to successfully treat pain, so with this in mind, a group of scientists and physicians at Mayo Clinic set out to study the effectiveness of acupuncture in the treatment of fibromyalgia symptoms.

To test this idea, the researchers took 50 patients who had been diagnosed with fibromyalgia and divided them into two groups of 25 each. All of them received the usual treatment for fibromyalgia at Mayo Clinic. From there, one group received true acupuncture, while the second group received a placebo — in this case, what's known as sham acupuncture (learn more about acupuncture research on the next page).

The research team achieved sham acupuncture first by placing a small stand in front of the patient's chest, so the patient couldn't see where the needles were being placed. Then, those who received sham acupuncture were given a brief poke by a toothpick without any skin penetration. An acupuncture needle, with its tip embedded into a bandage, was then placed over that point. That way, if a patient happened to look down, he or she would see the needle going through the bandage and believe that the needle also went through the skin.

Those who received true acupuncture also had the needle pass through a bandage, but in this case, it actually went into the skin. There is a fair amount of controversy over how best to create a placebo for acupuncture, but in terms of this study, when the patients were asked to guess whether they received true or sham acupuncture, about an equal number from each group guessed correctly, suggesting that the patients in the study were blind to the type of intervention they received.

In essence, all of the participants in this study were treated identically, with the only difference being that one group received eight treatments of true acupuncture. One month later, that group showed a statistically significant reduction in their Fibromyalgia Impact Questionnaire (FIQ) scores, a standard method of measuring fibromyalgia symptoms. These participants also felt less anxiety and pain. Six months later, the group that received true acupuncture still showed a statistically significant reduction in pain, anxiety and FIQ scores.

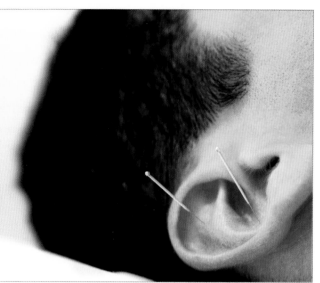

Our take

Acupuncture can be effective used alone, or when added to other medical treatments. The World Health Organization recognizes that acupuncture can be an effective treatment for a range of medical conditions.

Digestive disorders, such as constipation; respiratory disorders, such as allergic rhinitis; neurological and muscular disorders, such as headache, stroke and neck pain; low back pain and sciatica; and urinary and menstrual problems are among the medical conditions acupuncture may be able to help treat, according to medical experts and researchers.

What the research says

Acupuncture is difficult to truly study because in order to achieve a well-designed clinical trial, a placebo is needed. Research studies often use a sugar pill or saline injection for a placebo, but in acupuncture, it's more difficult to have a true placebo to test against.

Even with this challenge, and although acupuncture is still under study to determine exactly how it works from a scientific perspective, evidence shows that acupuncture is effective for certain conditions and certain people.

Pain

Treatment for pain is the best-studied aspect of acupuncture. The processing of pain signals involves many parts of the brain. In addition, how much pain you feel partly depends on the context.

Researchers at the University of Michigan found that acupuncture increases the number of opioid receptors in the brain. These structures play a key role in pain relief. The body's natural painkillers may play a key role in how acupuncture helps treat pain.

In addition, considerable evidence supports the idea that opioid peptides are released during acupuncture, and the pain-relieving effects of acupuncture are at least partially explained by their actions. Other research has shown that acupuncture can help treat a variety of different types of pain. Examples

include chronic neck pain, chronic and acute low back pain, knee pain, dental pain, osteoarthritis, labor pain, menstrual cramps, and headaches, including migraines.

Nausea and vomiting

Acupuncture can help reduce nausea and vomiting in people who are receiving chemotherapy. And although it isn't completely proved, some women find that acupuncture helps relieve morning sickness during pregnancy. Discuss using acupuncture during pregnancy to ensure that it's safe first (see page 96).

Spinal stenosis

Spinal stenosis is a painful arthritis of the lower spine in which the degenerative changes of the bones and joints impinge on the spinal cord or spinal nerves. Researchers evaluated acupuncture in patients with lumbar spinal stenosis and found significant improvement in pain intensity, overall symptoms and quality of life among those who received treatment compared with those who didn't.

However, the researchers couldn't say for certain that acupuncture was effective and safe for lumbar spinal stenosis because the research they studied was limited in scope and may have had a certain level of bias.

Herbs and supplements

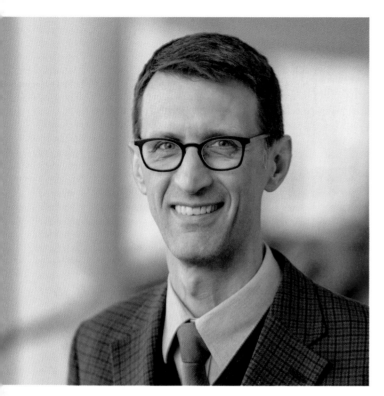

Jon C. Tilburt, M.D.
General Internal Medicine

Dr. Tilburt practices medicine as part of the integrative medicine program at Mayo Clinic in Rochester, Minnesota.

A visit with Dr. Tilburt

Dietary supplements are the most common form of integrative medicine used. With that said, when you're considering what role supplements can play in your overall wellness, remember this: *Dietary supplements are not a replacement for healthy lifestyle choices.* They are meant to supplement the healthy choices you make every day.

With this said, let's take a few minutes for a quick wellness tune-up, as I would have with one of my patients. Picture a three-legged stool. The seat of the stool represents how at peace you are with your life, a feeling I call well-being. The three legs represent nutrition, stress management and exercise. But don't forget about the floor underneath the stool. It's built from how well you're managing the symptoms you're experiencing. How strong and balanced does your wellness seat feel? Are there things you can do to make it more stable and secure?

There may be lifestyle choices you can make to strengthen the legs of your stool, which you read about earlier in this book. In addition, there may be integrative techniques, including supplements, that can help if you're having trouble managing a health condition. Supplements are one component of the nutritional leg of your wellness stool.

But what if you feel as if your wellness stool is sturdy and strong, and from a nutritional standpoint, you're already eating whole foods and plenty of vegetables? If this is the case, but you're still having trouble managing a health condition, then you may decide to explore supplements with your health care team. Bring up what you would like to accomplish and discuss what can help you reach your goals. Selected supplements can help nudge your body toward greater health.

In this section, you'll read about supplements that have been studied the most. If this section doesn't include a supplement you're interested in, visit the Additional resources part of this book (see page 214) for additional sources of information on supplements.

Safety first:
Being a smart supplement consumer

Herbs and other dietary supplements may be popular, but are they right for you? That depends on the product, your current health and your medical history.

Here's why: Dietary supplements contain ingredients that affect how your body functions, just as nonprescription and prescription medications do. Some supplements may be beneficial, but in other instances, herbal supplements may be risky. Their labels are often vague, and the supplements may pose more unwanted side effects than benefits. In some cases, they may even be dangerous for you — especially if you have certain allergies or if you take a medication that may interact with the supplement.

If you're considering a dietary supplement, take steps to get as much information as you can. This book is a good start, but other sources can help as well, including those listed in the Additional resources section of this book on page 214. Only take supplements that have undergone scientific testing to confirm their safety. And as with other integrative medicine therapies, talk to your doctor or another member of your health care team about any products you intend to use.

It's wise to avoid dietary supplements if:

You're pregnant or breast-feeding. As a general rule, don't take any medications when you're pregnant or breast-feeding unless your health care provider approves. Medications that may be safe for you as an adult may be harmful to your baby or your breast-feeding infant.

You're having surgery. Many herbal supplements can affect the success of surgery. Some may decrease the effectiveness of anesthetics or cause dangerous complications, such as bleeding or high blood pressure. Tell your doctor about any herbs you're taking as soon as you know you need surgery.

You're younger than 18 or older than 65. Older adults may metabolize medications differently than younger adults. And few herbal

supplements have been tested on children or have established safe doses for children.

While it's recommended that all individuals consult with a health care provider before taking dietary supplements, it's especially important that you do so if you take prescription or nonprescription medications. Some herbs can cause serious side effects, such as increased bleeding risk, when mixed with prescription or nonprescription drugs. Talk to your health care team about possible drug interactions. For more information on supplement safety, see page 199.

What a green light means

In upcoming pages, you'll find herbs and other supplements that have been given a green light. However, a green light does not always mean "go."

For instance, a green light doesn't mean it's OK to take the product for any condition or in any amount. Oftentimes, a product is given a green light because studies have found it is beneficial for just one or two conditions. There may be other conditions for which it isn't effective.

Always take supplements according to directions. Don't take more than is recommended, and always discuss your use of supplements with your health care provider. You'll note that the advice in this book generally includes a recommendation of not taking a product for more than six months. This is because — with some exceptions — most products haven't been studied for longer than six months to determine their long-term effects.

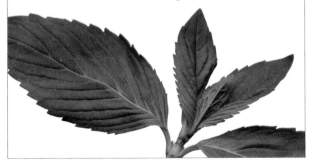

Expert insight

Supplements, then and now

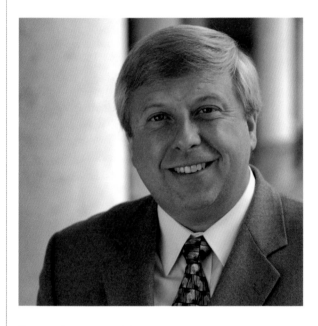

Brent A. Bauer, M.D.

Medical editor, *Mayo Clinic Guide to Integrative Medicine*

In addition to his role as a medical editor of this book, Dr. Bauer is director of research in Integrative Medicine and Health at Mayo Clinic in Rochester, Minnesota.

How has the use of supplements evolved during your 25 years at Mayo Clinic?

My interest in integrative medicine began at Mayo Clinic's campus in Arizona in 1992 as a newly minted staff physician. My first patient was a sweet 88-year-old woman holding a jar of echinacea and asking me what I thought about it.

None of my training had prepared me to answer her question — or the literally thousands of similar questions I would get over the years from other patients. As I looked for a way to approach the tough questions patients had, I realized that there were good and bad supplements and that good research was going to be the key in telling the difference between the two. Good research would also help me advise my patients on the safe and effective use of supplements as a partner in their quests to optimize their health.

In the last 25 years, there has been tremendous growth in research on supplements, which gives health care providers the means to provide helpful guidance on supplements.

Why does this book focus on a select group of supplements, rather than address all of the herbs and supplements on the market?

If we try to address the thousands of herbs and supplements and combinations on the shelves today, we'd have a 60-volume book that would need to be updated every six weeks to accommodate new research as it comes in.

Instead, we've chosen to focus on a select number of supplements that have strong research behind them so that we can provide the most useful information we can. With herbs, in particular, we've chosen to focus on those with broad appeal or common usage that have been studied enough that we can say more than, "more research is needed" — which is still the case for many.

Of the supplements your patients are using, which ones are offering the best results?

No one supplement is right for everybody. Deciding to take a supplement is a personal decision that's best made with your health care team after a thorough discussion of your personal circumstances and goals. With this said, there are several supplements that I'm seeing my patients take with good results.

For example, most of my patients are older and struggle with arthritis and inflammation. Many of them are able to ease their symptoms more effectively by adding fish oil to their overall approach to managing arthritis. Along the same lines, other supplements my patients are using with good results include probiotics, vitamin D, curcumin, SAMe, glucosamine, chondroitin, coenzyme Q10, American ginseng and ginger.

Herbs and supplements

Fish oil

Fish oil is one of the most widely used dietary supplements in the United States. It's been studied for heart health since it was found that the Inuit people of North America have a lower risk of heart disease even though they eat a high-fat diet.

Fish oil is a source of omega-3 fatty acids — substances your body needs to perform many functions, from muscle activity to cell growth. Omega-3 fatty acids are derived from food. They cannot be manufactured in the body.

Fish oil contains two omega-3s called docosahexaenoic acid (DHA) and eicosapentaenoic acid (EPA). Dietary sources of DHA and EPA are fatty fish (salmon, mackerel and trout) and shellfish (mussels, oysters and crabs). Some nuts, seeds and vegetable oils contain another omega-3 called alpha-linolenic acid (ALA).

Omega-3 fatty acids have been shown to improve cardiovascular health, helping to reduce the risk of heart attack, stroke, high triglycerides and high blood pressure. They also appear to improve symptoms of rheumatoid arthritis.

Fish oil supplements, which come in liquid, capsule and pill form, are generally safe when used as recommended. Most people can take 3 grams (3,000 milligrams) a day without experiencing adverse effects.

Our take

Omega-3 fatty acids are essential for good health, but try to get them from your diet by eating broiled or baked fish. Fish oil supplements may be best suited for individuals with heart disease or an autoimmune disorder. Fish oil supplements are generally safe — though high doses can be harmful. Too much fish oil can increase your risk of bleeding and may suppress your immune response. Take fish oil supplements under a doctor's supervision.

What the research says

Heart disease

While study results have been mixed, there is evidence that fish oil supplements are effective for heart disease.

Research shows that eating dietary sources of fish oil — such as tuna or salmon — twice a week is associated with a reduced risk of developing heart disease. And taking fish oil supplements for at least six months has been shown to reduce the risk of heart-related events (such as heart attack) and death in people who are at high risk of heart disease. Research also suggests that the risk of congestive heart failure is lower in older adults who have higher levels of EPA fatty acids.

High blood pressure

Multiple studies report modest reductions in blood pressure in people who take fish oil supplements. There is some evidence that this effect is greater for people with moderate to severe hypertension than those with mild hypertension.

Lipids

There's strong evidence that omega-3 fatty acids can significantly reduce blood triglyceride levels. There also appears to be a slight improvement in high-density lipoprotein (HDL), or "good," cholesterol, although an increase in levels of low-density lipoprotein (LDL), or "bad," cholesterol also was observed.

Rheumatoid arthritis

Studies suggest fish oil supplements may help reduce pain, improve morning stiffness and relieve joint tenderness in people with rheumatoid arthritis. While relief is often modest, it may be enough to reduce the need for anti-inflammatory medications.

Glucosamine and chondroitin

Glucosamine and chondroitin are natural compounds found in cartilage — the tough tissue that cushions joints. These supplements are used to treat a painful condition caused by the inflammation, breakdown and eventual loss of cartilage (osteoarthritis).

There are several forms of glucosamine. The form considered best suited for cartilage repair is glucosamine sulfate. Glucosamine is often administered with chondroitin to treat osteoarthritis.

When considering glucosamine and chondroitin, read product labels carefully. Avoid confusing glucosamine sulfate with N-acetylglucosamine. Glucosamine sulfate has been studied for treatment of arthritis; however, there's no clinical evidence to support the use of N-acetylglucosamine in treating arthritis.

Glucosamine and chondroitin appear to be safe and to produce few side effects. However, if you're allergic to shellfish, it's generally best to avoid them. Use caution if you take an anticoagulant drug, such as warfarin (Coumadin, Jantoven). Glucosamine may increase the risk of bleeding.

Our take

Glucosamine and chondroitin have become a popular treatment for osteoarthritis.

They appear to be safe and produce fewer adverse side effects than do medications such as nonsteroidal anti-inflammatory drugs (NSAIDs).

But how effective are glucosamine and chondroitin at treating arthritis? Many older studies gave promising results. However, a few recent studies question whether these supplements actually make a difference.

For instance, results from a large trial sponsored by the National Institutes of Health were mostly negative. The only individuals who appeared to receive some benefit were those with very severe symptoms.

While study results are mixed, side effects from the supplements are few and far between. So far, no other treatments have shown promise in increasing cartilage. And it's still possible glucosamine and chondroitin may help. Therefore, they may be worth a try.

What the research says

Osteoarthritis

There is conflicting evidence about the effect of glucosamine and chondroitin on osteoarthritis.

Some research shows that glucosamine and chondroitin can help decrease pain and improve joint function in people who have osteoarthritis. For instance, one European study suggested that glucosamine was more effective than acetaminophen (Tylenol, others) in reducing joint pain from osteoarthritis. And an analysis of 17 published trials concluded that glucosamine sulfate might delay the progression and help symptoms of knee osteoarthritis. These are all promising findings.

Unfortunately, there are also some not-so-promising results, as well. The National Institutes of Health (NIH) sponsored a study in which glucosamine and chondroitin were used to treat osteoarthritis of the knee. Results of the study suggested that — when given separately or in combination — glucosamine and chondroitin weren't any more effective in treating pain than was an inactive substance (placebo). The study also didn't find glucosamine and chondroitin to slow cartilage loss. And a 2015 study of people with knee osteoarthritis didn't find significant pain improvement from glucosamine and chondroitin.

Rheumatoid arthritis

Evidence for glucosamine and chondroitin's effect on rheumatoid arthritis is limited, but early research suggests that glucosamine may reduce RA-related pain when compared with a placebo. However, researchers didn't see an improvement in inflammation or the number of painful or swollen joints. More research is needed.

Probiotics and prebiotics

The term *probiotics* refers to dietary supplements or foods that contain beneficial, or "good," bacteria similar to those normally found in the body. A common probiotic bacterium is *Lactobacillus acidophilus*.

Good bacteria compete with and offer protection from harmful, disease-causing bacteria — just as the existing good bacteria in your body already do. Probiotic bacteria help maintain a proper microorganic balance in your intestinal tract, and also help with digestion.

Prebiotics are nondigestible carbohydrates that act as food for probiotics. When probiotics and prebiotics are combined, they form synbiotics.

Probiotics come from food sources such as yogurt, cheese, miso, tempeh, and some juices and soy drinks. Prebiotics are found in whole grains, bananas, onions, garlic, honey and artichokes. As supplements, they're available as capsules, tablets, suppositories and powders. They may also be added to some foods.

Researchers have studied probiotics to find out whether they might help prevent or treat a variety of health problems, such as digestive problems, allergies, eczema, oral health conditions, colic in babies and yeast infections.

Probiotics and prebiotics are generally safe for healthy people. Side effects, if they occur, tend to be mild. Gas and bloating are the most common. In some people with serious medical problems — such as those who have weakened immune systems — probiotics may deliver serious side effects, including dangerous infections.

Our take

There's growing interest in probiotics, spurred by their potential to treat various gastrointestinal disorders. While some probiotics have shown encouraging results in studies, more research is needed. In the meantime, there appears to be little harm in taking supplements, although a good, balanced diet generally should provide you with enough good bacteria.

What the research says

Cold and flu
There's good evidence that probiotics can reduce the risk of contracting the common cold and the flu, and reduce the severity of symptoms. However, more research is needed to confirm these findings.

Diarrhea
Studies suggest that probiotic supplements may be effective in reducing the risk and duration of both viral diarrhea and diarrhea following antibiotic treatment. Probiotics may also reduce your risk of developing traveler's diarrhea. More research is needed to determine which probiotics may be most effective for managing diarrhea.

Eczema
Probiotics seem to reduce the severity of eczema (atopic dermatitis) in infants and children.

Irritable bowel syndrome
Research suggests that probiotics may be helpful for managing the symptoms of irritable bowel syndrome. However, more research is needed.

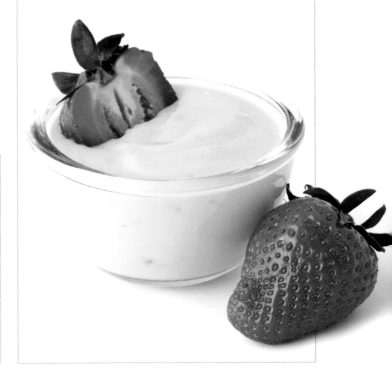

Melatonin

Melatonin is a hormone that occurs naturally in your body to control the internal system that regulates when you fall asleep and when you wake up (circadian rhythm). The production and release of melatonin is connected to time of day, increasing when it's dark and decreasing when it's light. Levels in the blood are highest just before bedtime.

Melatonin also helps control the release of female reproductive hormones, which determines the timing of the menstrual cycles and menopause.

Melatonin supplements — which are available as tablets, capsules, creams and lozenges — are created from the amino acid tryptophan. Although they are used for a variety of medical conditions, they are most notably used for disorders related to sleep, such as insomnia and jet lag. Melatonin is also advertised as a treatment for other conditions, such as arthritis, stress, migraines, heart disease, dementia and cancer.

Our take

Melatonin can promote sleep and appears to be safe for short-term use, but its long-term safety is unknown. It's likely that your body produces enough melatonin for its general needs, and taking supplements regularly isn't needed. Melatonin may be used occasionally, such as to get your wake-sleep cycle back on track when you have jet lag. In general, treat melatonin as you would any form of sleeping pill, and use it under your doctor's supervision.

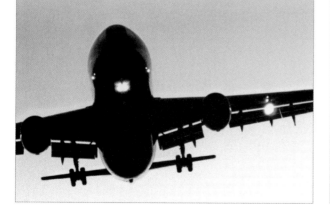

What the research says

Insomnia
Research suggests that melatonin may provide relief from the inability to fall asleep and stay asleep (insomnia) by slightly improving your total sleep time, sleep quality and how long it takes you to fall asleep. However, more research is needed. Little is known of the long-term effects, or how melatonin compares with insomnia medications.

Jet lag
Studies indicate that melatonin, when taken on the day of travel and continued for several days, may help ease the daytime fatigue and sleep disturbances associated with jet lag, and reduce the time required to re-establish a normal sleep pattern. However, the symptoms of jet lag are variable and not always easy to assess.

Sleep enhancement
Several studies indicate that healthy individuals who take melatonin before bedtime will fall asleep faster. It's unknown whether it will help people stay asleep.

Delayed sleep phase disorder
Studies suggest that melatonin may be able to help correct the sleep-wake rhythm in a condition in which the sleep-wake cycle is delayed by three to six hours (delayed sleep phase disorder).

Shift work disorder
Research suggests that melatonin may improve daytime sleep quality and duration for people whose jobs require them to work outside the traditional morning to evening schedule.

Other uses
Melatonin has been studied as a treatment for cancer, headache, seasonal affective disorder and smoking cessation. Recent research also is exploring whether melatonin may play a role in improving facets of Alzheimer's disease and amyotrophic lateral sclerosis (ALS). Melatonin may also play a role in sleep disorders associated with menopause, depression and schizophrenia. More research is needed in these areas.

Coenzyme Q10

Coenzyme Q10 (CoQ10) is an antioxidant that your body produces naturally. CoQ10 produces energy for cell development and maintenance — and is an essential part of your body's basic cell function.

The levels of CoQ10 in your body decrease as you age. CoQ10 levels have also been found to be lower in people with certain conditions, including heart disease, Parkinson's disease, diabetes and some cancers.

Although your body manufactures CoQ10, you can find it in certain foods, as well. Examples include meat, fish and whole grains. The amount of CoQ10 found in these dietary sources, however, isn't enough to significantly increase CoQ10 levels in your body.

CoQ10 may help treat disorders such as heart disease, high blood pressure, asthma, migraines, Parkinson's disease and certain cancers. It's also believed to help prevent aging effects and memory loss, and to improve exercise performance.

CoQ10 supplements appear to be safe and to produce very few side effects when taken as directed. Mild side effects may include nausea, headaches, insomnia, fatigue, dizziness and irritability. You generally shouldn't use CoQ10 if you're pregnant or breast-feeding. And talk to your doctor before using CoQ10 if you take an anticoagulant medication, such as warfarin (Coumadin, Jantoven), as it may make it less effective.

Our take

CoQ10 gets a green light because the supplements may be beneficial for treating conditions such as congestive heart failure, high blood pressure and Parkinson's disease. They may also help prevent a condition that can arise from use of statin cholesterol medications (statin-induced myopathy).

CoQ10 is also considered safe, with only minor, if any, side effects. However, it is wise to take this supplement under your health care provider's supervision.

What the research says

Heart (cardiovascular) conditions

While studies have produced mixed results, research does suggest that CoQ10 supplements may be effective for cardiovascular conditions. CoQ10 may help cause a decrease in blood pressure and improve symptoms of congestive heart failure. CoQ10 may also be effective for improving heart function to help prevent future cardiovascular disease. Preliminary research also suggests that when combined with other nutrients, CoQ10 may aid recovery in people who've had bypass and heart valve surgeries. More research is necessary to confirm CoQ10's effects on heart conditions.

Migraines

CoQ10 is also being studied as a treatment for migraines. Preliminary research suggests that CoQ10 may help prevent and decrease the frequency of these headaches.

Parkinson's disease

Preliminary studies suggest that CoQ10 may slow decline and improve symptoms of Parkinson's disease. More research is needed.

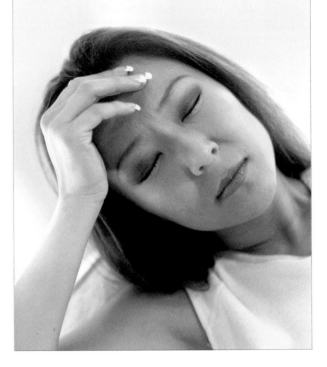

Vitamin D

Your body manufactures vitamin D when direct sunlight converts a chemical in your skin into an active form of the vitamin (calciferol). Vitamin D is necessary for building and maintaining healthy bones. That's because calcium, the primary component of bone, can only be absorbed by your body when vitamin D is present.

Vitamin D is not found in many foods, but you can get it from a few dietary sources. These include fortified milk, fortified cereal, and fatty fish such as salmon, mackerel and sardines.

The amount of vitamin D your skin makes depends on many factors, including the time of day, season, latitude of the region where you live and your skin pigmentation. Depending on where you live and your lifestyle, vitamin D production may decrease or be completely absent during the winter months. Sunscreen, while important, also can decrease vitamin D production.

The current recommended daily allowance for vitamin D developed by the Food and Nutrition Board is 400 international units (IU) for children up to age 12 months, 600 IU for ages 1 to 70 years, and 800 IU for people over 70 years. As a point of reference, an 8-oz. glass of milk provides about 115 to 124 IU and 3 ounces of salmon provides nearly 450 IU.

Our take

Vitamin D is essential to your health. Without it, your bones can become soft, thin and brittle — a condition known as osteomalacia. Insufficient vitamin D is connected to other conditions, as well, including osteoporosis and some types of cancer.

If you do not get enough vitamin D through sunlight or dietary sources, supplements may be necessary. In unusual circumstances, some people may need very high doses of vitamin D. But in most circumstances, taking more than 4,000 IU a day appears to increase the risk of side effects, including confusion, heart rhythm problems and kidney damage.

What the research says

Cancer
Research suggests that vitamin D, especially when taken with calcium, may help prevent certain cancers. However, further research is needed.

Cognitive health
Early research suggests that vitamin D may play a role in cognitive health. In one small study of adults age 60 years and older who were being treated for dementia, researchers found that taking a vitamin D supplement helped improve cognitive function.

Falls
Research shows that older adults who get adequate amounts of vitamin D on a daily basis experience fewer falls.

Inherited disorders
Vitamin D supplements can be used to help treat inherited disorders resulting from an inability to absorb or process vitamin D, such as familial hypophosphatemia.

Osteomalacia
Vitamin D supplements are used to treat adults with severe vitamin D deficiency, resulting in loss of bone mineral content, bone pain, muscle weakness and soft bones (osteomalacia).

Osteoporosis
Studies suggest that people who get enough vitamin D and calcium in their diets can slow bone mineral loss, help prevent osteoporosis and reduce bone fractures.

Psoriasis
Applying vitamin D or a topical preparation that contains a vitamin D compound called calcipotriene (Dovonex) to the skin can treat plaque-type psoriasis in some people.

Rickets
This rare condition develops in children with vitamin D deficiency. Supplementing with vitamin D can prevent and treat the problem.

Echinacea

You may know echinacea by its common name, the coneflower. It belongs to the same plant family as the sunflower, thistle and black-eyed Susan.

The roots and herbs from three echinacea species (*Echinacea purpurea*, *Echinacea angustifolia*, and *Echinacea pallida*) may be used in pills, teas or juices, extracts, or external applications. The most popular is *Echinacea purpurea*, also known as the Eastern purple coneflower.

Echinacea traditionally has been used to treat many conditions, from skin wounds and acne to dizziness and cancer. Starting in the 20th century, echinacea became a popular remedy for colds, flu and upper respiratory tract infections. This more recent interest is due to echinacea's purported ability to boost the immune system to more effectively fight infection.

While the bulk of echinacea research has been focused on upper respiratory infections, the plant has also been studied for its potential effects on tonsillitis, anxiety, gingivitis and other conditions in recent years.

Because the active ingredient in echinacea hasn't been identified, there's often a problem with quality control. Some products may contain very small amounts of echinacea, if any at all.

Our take

Unfortunately, there's still no cure for the common cold. Despite all of the claims, the latest research suggests echinacea isn't an effective method for prevention or treatment of upper respiratory infections, as once thought. While some studies have found modest benefits, echinacea hasn't been found to deliver significant decreases in the length or severity of colds.

If you have a cold, it won't hurt you to try echinacea for a few days, but there's no guarantee that it will help. Don't use it for more than eight weeks at a time. But if you're allergic to plants in the daisy family, beware of allergic reactions, including anaphylaxis.

As for echinacea's other claims, the research isn't there yet. It's unclear whether echinacea can boost the immune system.

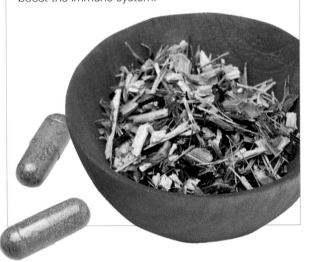

What the research says

Cancer
There's no clear evidence that echinacea has an effect on any type of cancer in humans. However, some research suggests that echinacea may help improve red and white blood cell counts during chemotherapy treatment in women with advanced breast cancer.

Gingivitis
Research suggests that echinacea may slightly reduce inflammation associated with the gum disease gingivitis. More research is needed.

Immune system
Echinacea has been studied alone and in combination with other ingredients for its effect on the immune system. It's still unclear if there are any significant benefits.

Upper respiratory tract infections
The debate continues about whether echinacea can treat or prevent the common cold and other upper respiratory tract infections. While several well-respected studies have found echinacea to be of little to no benefit, other studies suggest that echinacea may reduce the duration and severity of upper respiratory infections, or even reduce the risk of getting a cold. More research is needed.

Black cohosh

Black cohosh (*Actaea racemosa or Cimicifuga racemosa*) is a member of the buttercup family. The underground stems (rhizomes) and roots of black cohosh are commonly used fresh or dried to make strong teas, capsules, and solid or liquid extracts.

Black cohosh was originally used in Native American medicine, and was a home remedy for rheumatic joint pain and arthritis in 19th-century America. It was later discovered that black cohosh has effects similar to the female hormone estrogen. As a result, in recent years, black cohosh has become popular for treating hot flashes, night sweats, vaginal dryness, headaches and other menopausal symptoms. It's also been used for premenstrual pain and menstrual irregularities and to induce labor.

Black cohosh is generally well-tolerated. Mild side effects may include stomach discomfort, headache or rash.

For the most part, studies haven't found black cohosh to cause serious side effects. However, it's generally best not to take black cohosh for longer than six months or during pregnancy. Also, there is some concern it may cause liver damage in some people. Do not take black cohosh if you have a liver disorder.

Our take

While some research suggests that black cohosh may improve menopausal symptoms, there just isn't enough evidence to make a definitive recommendation. Study results are mixed, with some trials finding encouraging results and other trials failing to return promising data. However, if you're experiencing bothersome menopausal symptoms, you may consider trying black cohosh to see if it works for you, especially given the fact that hormone therapy is no longer an option for most women. Don't use it for more than six months at a time, and talk to your health care team if you notice any troubling side effects.

For other conditions, there's less evidence black cohosh may be beneficial, so be cautious.

What the research says

Menopausal symptoms
There is conflicting research on black cohosh's effect on menopausal symptoms. While some studies suggest that black cohosh may help relieve hot flashes, headaches and other menopausal symptoms, other studies do not. In fact, one review of six clinical trials for the relief of menopausal symptoms found that black cohosh, whether used alone or with other botanicals, failed to relieve hot flashes and night sweats in postmenopausal women or those approaching menopause.

Research is ongoing to determine the potential effects of black cohosh on menopausal symptoms and how this supplement might improve quality of life during menopause.

Rheumatism
There is not enough reliable evidence to determine whether black cohosh is effective at relieving the pain and inflammation of rheumatism.

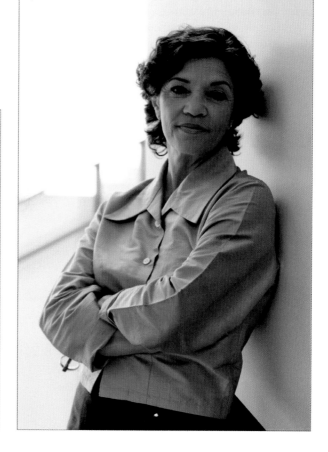

Saw palmetto

Saw palmetto (*Serenoa repens*) is a small palm tree that thrives in the United States' warm southeastern climate. It's also called the American dwarf palm tree, and cabbage palm.

The plant's dark purple berries were a staple food of American Indians. As a supplement, saw palmetto is available as a liquid extract, tablet, capsule and as an infusion or a tea.

Many products containing saw palmetto, frequently in combination with other ingredients, are on the market today. In Europe, saw palmetto is popularly used to treat the urinary symptoms associated with an enlarged prostate gland, a condition called benign prostatic hyperplasia (BPH). Although saw palmetto is often recommended for BPH as an alternative medicine in the United States, it's not considered a standard treatment.

Saw palmetto may also be used as a diuretic, an antiseptic and a sedative, as well as for chronic pelvic pain, bladder disorders, decreased sex drive, hormone imbalances and prostate cancer.

When taken in recommended doses, saw palmetto is generally well-tolerated. However, avoid using this supplement if you're pregnant or lactating, as it can affect your hormones.

Our take

In some men, saw palmetto can be an effective treatment for managing symptoms of an enlarged prostate. Study results have been mixed. While some studies have found saw palmetto to be modestly effective for treating BPH, others have found it to be of no benefit. Because saw palmetto is generally safe, it doesn't hurt to give it a try.

Don't use saw palmetto if you have a bleeding problem because there is some evidence that it can increase bleeding.

As with other supplements, talk to your health care team before using saw palmetto.

What the research says

More research is necessary to evaluate saw palmetto for the conditions for which it's most popular. Here's what the most recent studies have to say about saw palmetto:

Benign prostatic hyperplasia (BPH)

Several small studies suggest that saw palmetto may be effective for treating BPH symptoms, such as poor urine flow, inflammation and frequent nighttime urination. However, other studies — including a reputable 2011 study of 369 older men — showed that saw palmetto didn't reduce BPH-related urinary symptoms more than an inactive substance (placebo). More research needs to be done to determine whether saw palmetto is effective for this use.

Prostate cancer

Research suggests that taking saw palmetto does not lower the risk of developing prostate cancer.

Other uses

While saw palmetto has been studied for its effects on other conditions, such as prostate-specific antigen (PSA) levels, pelvic pain, bladder disorders and hair loss, there is not enough reliable evidence to rate its effectiveness. More research is needed.

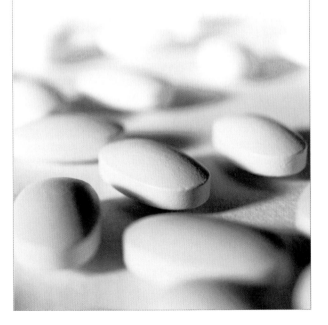

Garlic

Garlic (*Allium sativum*) has been used for centuries to treat conditions ranging from high blood pressure to protection from snake venom. Researchers believe the compound allicin, which gives garlic its aroma and flavor, is responsible for garlic's health benefits. Allicin is thought to be a powerful antioxidant.

Garlic is most effective when you eat the bulb raw, but it can also be purchased cut, ground, dried or powdered, and in tablet or capsule form. Garlic can also be used to make oils and liquid extracts.

Garlic's most common uses are for high cholesterol, heart disease and high blood pressure. It may also be used to prevent certain cancers, including stomach and colon cancer.

Garlic is safe for most adults. Side effects are typically mild, and may include breath and body odor. Heartburn and upset stomach may occur if taken on an empty stomach.

Talk to your health care provider about possible drug interactions before taking garlic, since it can interfere with some prescription medications. Because garlic can reduce the ability of the blood to clot, it may increase your risk of bleeding if you take anticoagulant medications. Garlic may also decrease the effectiveness of contraceptives. And because garlic may lower your blood pressure, it may not be safe to take with antihypertensive medications. Other medications, including the HIV medication saquinavir, may pose serious interactions when taken with garlic.

Our take

Garlic gets a green light because studies suggest that garlic and garlic supplements may help lower low-density lipoprotein (LDL), or "bad," cholesterol, and contribute to heart health. The supplements appear to be of low risk, except in individuals taking certain medications.

If you take garlic tablets, make sure they contain *allicin*, garlic's active ingredient. Odor-free preparations may not include allicin.

What the research says

Cancer
Some studies suggest consuming garlic as a regular part of your diet may lower the risk of certain cancers, including stomach and colon cancers. However, other studies, such as those on lung and breast cancer, have not found decreased risks. More research needs to be done to confirm all findings.

Cholesterol
While some research on garlic's effect on cholesterol is promising, results are mixed. Early research found small reductions in total blood cholesterol and in low-density lipoprotein (LDL), or "bad," cholesterol from garlic use. Other, more recent, studies have found garlic to be less effective at lowering cholesterol levels. Further research is needed to gather more information.

Heart
Garlic may have heart-healthy benefits. Research suggests garlic may slow hardening of the arteries, a condition that can lead to heart disease. And there is evidence that garlic may also reduce blood pressure in people with hypertension, a condition that can lead to heart problems.

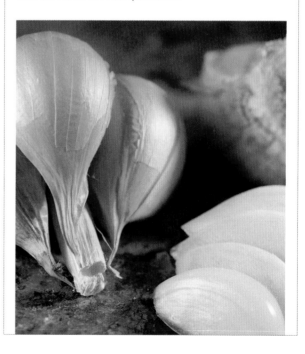

Ginkgo

Ginkgo (*Ginkgo biloba*) is one of the oldest living species of tree. Its fan-shaped leaves and its seeds have both been used in traditional medicine for thousands of years. Ginkgo is most commonly available as a tablet, capsule or tea.

The most helpful components of ginkgo are believed to be flavonoids, which have powerful antioxidant qualities, and terpenoids, which help improve circulation by dilating blood vessels and reducing the "stickiness" of platelets.

Ginkgo has been studied for a wide range of conditions, from anxiety to cognitive function. Most research, however, has focused on ginkgo's effect on dementia, memory impairment and leg pain caused by narrowing arteries (claudication).

Ginkgo has been used to treat circulatory disorders and symptoms associated with reduced blood flow to the brain, particularly in older adults. These symptoms include memory loss, dizziness, headache and ringing in the ears (tinnitus).

When taken in recommended doses, ginkgo is generally well-tolerated. Mild side effects may include nausea, stomach upset, headache, dizziness, diarrhea and allergic skin reactions. There is some concern that ginkgo may increase bleeding risk, so talk to your health care provider if you have a bleeding disorder or take an anticoagulant medication such as warfarin (Coumadin, Jantoven). And don't take ginkgo during pregnancy, as it may have hormonal and labor-inducing effects.

Our take

Studies have produced some encouraging results for the use of ginkgo as a treatment for certain circulation disorders and what are sometimes called cerebral insufficiencies — symptoms such as absent-mindedness and confusion — which may be associated with Alzheimer's disease. However, studies have found ginkgo isn't an overall "brain booster," as once thought, and its effectiveness hasn't been proved.

What the research says

Claudication
Some studies suggest that ginkgo causes small improvements in the symptoms of claudication, such as leg pain due to clogged arteries. However, ginkgo may not be as helpful for this condition as exercise or some prescription drugs.

Dementia
Some early studies suggested that ginkgo improved symptoms of early-stage Alzheimer's disease and certain dementias. In fact, a study in 2000 found a ginkgo extract to be as helpful as some drugs. But more recent studies, which have been larger and well-controlled, indicate that ginkgo doesn't reduce the risk or progression of Alzheimer's or other dementias.

Memory enhancement
Ginkgo's effect on memory enhancement has also had conflicting results. While some evidence suggests that ginkgo extract may modestly improve memory in healthy adults, most studies indicate that ginkgo doesn't improve memory, attention and brain function.

Tinnitus
Although some studies have delivered positive results, most evidence suggests that ginkgo does not improve symptoms of ringing in the ears (tinnitus).

Other uses
Studies indicate possible benefits of ginkgo in the treatment of anxiety, diabetic retinopathy, schizophrenia, vertigo, seasonal affective disorder, glaucoma, macular degeneration, sexual dysfunction, and some symptoms of premenstrual syndrome (PMS). More research needs to be conducted to determine whether ginkgo is an effective treatment for these conditions.

Turmeric

Turmeric (*Curcuma longa*) is a plant that is grown in India, Asia and Africa. Its trademark golden color makes it a popular fabric dye, and its mild but distinctive taste makes it a common ingredient in many Indian and Asian dishes, such as curry powders and flavored rices.

Similar to its relative, the ginger plant, the part of the turmeric plant used in spices and supplements is the underground stem (rhizome). Turmeric is available as a powder, capsule, tea or extract. In some cases, it's made into a paste to apply to the skin.

Traditional uses of turmeric are many, and range from relieving joint pain to regulating menstruation. Turmeric has also been used on the skin for eczema, for itchiness and to help wounds heal. More recently, uses include treating inflammation, heartburn, gallstones and cancer.

Our take

Although turmeric has been used for thousands of years in India and Asia, relatively little scientific research has been conducted to support its use for health conditions.

Some studies suggest that turmeric — and, more specifically, a chemical found in turmeric called curcumin — may be an effective treatment for pain, inflammation, high cholesterol and other medical conditions, but more research is necessary to confirm these findings.

For most adults, turmeric is safe to use — so there's no harm in trying it to see if it works for you. Side effects are usually mild, though there is some evidence that high doses or long-term use may cause indigestion, nausea or diarrhea.

Ask your health care provider about taking turmeric if you have gallbladder disease, since it may worsen the condition, or if you take an anticoagulant medication, such as warfarin, as turmeric may increase the risk of bleeding.

What the research says

High cholesterol
Some research suggests that turmeric supplements may be effective in reducing cholesterol and triglyceride levels. In one study, overweight people with a high level of fats, or lipids, in the blood (hyperlipidemia) experienced a decrease in total cholesterol, low-density lipoprotein (LDL), or "bad," cholesterol and triglycerides, a type of fat found in your blood.

Osteoarthritis
Several studies on turmeric's relation to osteoarthritis have been conducted. Research suggests that turmeric may reduce pain and increase ease of movement in people with this condition. In fact, when it comes to pain relief, one study found that taking turmeric extract three times daily was comparable to taking 1,200 milligrams of ibuprofen daily. While these results are promising, more research is necessary.

Rheumatoid arthritis
Some evidence suggests that turmeric might lessen some of the symptoms of rheumatoid arthritis, such as joint swelling and morning stiffness. More research is needed to confirm these findings.

Other uses
Turmeric's effect on Alzheimer's disease, Crohn's disease, certain cancers (including colorectal and prostate), depression, diabetes, joint pain, irritable bowel syndrome and other conditions is also being explored.

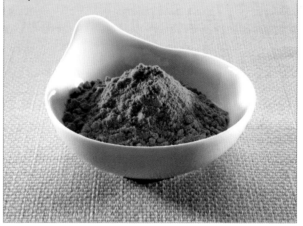

Ginseng

The term *ginseng* is associated with 13 different species of perennial, deciduous plants in the genus *Panax*. As a supplement, however, ginseng most commonly refers to Asian ginseng (*Panax ginseng*) and sometimes refers to American ginseng (*Panax quinquefolius*).

Asian ginseng grows in China, Korea and Siberia. The gnarled, brown ginseng root is the part of the plant that's used in supplements. Ginseng root sometimes resembles a human body because of the stringy offshoots that look like arms and legs. Due to that resemblance, practitioners of traditional Chinese medicine often considered the herb a cure-all for most human ills, including: allergies, asthma, appetite stimulant, bleeding disorders, breathing difficulties, cancer, dizziness, headache, heart disorders, insomnia, liver disease, stroke and many more. Asian ginseng has been used for health-related purposes for more than 2,000 years.

Ginseng is considered safe when taken for short periods. Side effects, if any, tend to be mild and include headaches and sleep and gastrointestinal problems.

However, don't use ginseng for more than six months or exceed the recommended maximum daily doses. Also, avoid taking ginseng if you're pregnant, as some research suggests it could contribute to birth defects.

Our take

Evidence suggests that short-term use of ginseng may improve mental performance and that it produces few side effects when taken as directed. Therefore, ginseng gets a green light. However, do not take ginseng for an extended period of time. More research is needed before specific recommendations regarding its use can be made.

More studies are also needed to determine how effective ginseng is in terms of other conditions such as cancer and diabetes.

What the research says

Cancer
Some evidence suggests that ginseng may improve quality of life for those who have cancer. Results are mixed, however, for ginseng's effect on cancer risk. Some preliminary studies suggest that ginseng may reduce the risk of certain cancers, while other research contradicts these findings. More research is necessary.

Erectile dysfunction
Research suggests that ginseng may improve sexual function in men who have erectile dysfunction.

Exercise performance
Some athletes use ginseng to improve stamina, but it's unclear whether it provides any benefit. Research does suggest that ginseng does not improve aerobic performance. More research is necessary.

Heart
Ginseng appears to have some antioxidant effects that may benefit people with heart disorders. However, better studies are needed to make a firm recommendation.

Mental performance and mood
Studies report that ginseng may modestly improve mood, reaction times, and thinking, attention and learning performance in healthy middle-aged people. There is also some evidence that — while ginseng does not appear to improve memory — it may have a positive effect on cognitive performance in people with Alzheimer's disease. More research is needed.

Type 2 diabetes
Evidence for ginseng's effect on type 2 diabetes is mixed. Some studies report that ginseng may lower blood sugar levels in people with type 2 diabetes, while other studies suggest that ginseng does not significantly improve glucose concentrations. More research is needed.

St. John's wort

St. John's wort (*Hypericum perforatum*) is a flowering shrub native to Europe. It gets its name from the fact that it's often in full bloom on the traditional date of the birthday of the biblical John the Baptist. It has a long history as a treatment for depression, anxiety, insomnia and nervous disorders. It's also prepared as a salve for wounds and burns.

The flowers and leaves of St. John's wort contain active ingredients such as hyperforin. But there are other, still unidentified but active, components in the plant. St. John's wort is available in teas, tablets, powders and liquids. Topical preparations are also available.

Although St. John's wort is believed to be safe for general use, it does come with potential side effects. People who take St. John's wort may experience gastrointestinal upset and increased sensitivity to sunlight. A more serious concern, however, is the potential for drug interactions. Some of the active compounds in St. John's wort don't mix well with prescription drugs and other supplements. These include antidepressant medications, birth control pills, anticoagulant drugs, seizure-control drugs, certain asthma medications and steroids. These cautions make it especially important that you talk to your health care team before using St. John's wort.

Our take

St. John's wort can be effective for treating mild to moderate depression, and it's relatively safe. Its drawback — and the reason we give it a yellow light instead of a green light — is that it interacts with many medications and has caused serious side effects. In general, don't take St. John's wort if you take prescription medications.

St. John's wort also hasn't been proved safe to use during pregnancy. And it may increase your skin's sensitivity to sunlight. For all of these reasons, it's important to talk to your health care provider before taking St. John's wort.

What the research says

Studies on St. John's wort have generally focused on depression and anxiety. Here's what the latest research shows.

Anxiety

While anecdotal evidence suggests that St. John's wort may help relieve symptoms of anxiety, scientific studies have found mixed results. In one study, St. John's wort was combined with the herb valerian to reduce moderate to severe anxiety. However, there's not enough evidence to make a recommendation at this time.

Depression

Several studies support the therapeutic benefit of St. John's wort in treating mild to moderate depression. In fact, some research has shown the supplement to be as effective as several prescription antidepressants and with fewer side effects.

Despite these positive results, St. John's wort is not a proven treatment for depression. Two studies have reported no benefits for major depression. The greatest concern with using St. John's wort is the potential for serious interactions with various types of prescription drugs.

As with other supplements, do not use St. John's wort in place of conventional care — or without consulting with your health care provider.

Menopausal symptoms

Some evidence suggests that taking St. John's wort combined with a particular form of black cohosh extract may reduce menopausal symptoms, such as hot flashes. The research is less compelling when St. John's wort is used alone. While some studies suggest St. John's wort may reduce the frequency and severity of hot flashes, other studies do not. More research is necessary.

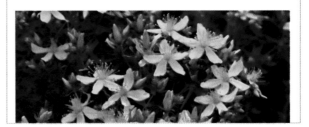

Flaxseed and flaxseed oil

Flaxseed (*Linum usitatissimum*) can be used whole or crushed, or in a powder form as meal or flour. Flaxseed oil, which comes from flaxseeds, is available in liquid and capsule form.

Flaxseed and flaxseed oil are used to lower cholesterol and blood sugar and treat many digestive conditions. Some people take flaxseed to treat inflammatory diseases. Flaxseed, but not flaxseed oil, is also used to relieve menopausal symptoms.

Both flaxseed and flaxseed oil are rich sources of alpha-linolenic acid, one of the heart-healthy omega-3 fatty acids. Flaxseed is also high in soluble fiber and in lignans — which contain phytoestrogens. It's believed that phytoestrogens, which are similar to the hormone estrogen, may have anti-cancer properties. Flaxseed oil does not have these phytoestrogens.

Flaxseed and flaxseed oil are generally safe to use in recommended doses. However, when taken in large amounts and with too little water, flaxseed may cause digestive issues, such as bloating, gas or diarrhea.

In general, don't take flaxseed at the same time as medications or other dietary supplements, because it may lower your body's ability to absorb them. And it's best to avoid flaxseed and flaxseed oil when you're pregnant.

Our take

When flaxseed is consumed as part of a healthy lifestyle approach — an approach that also includes daily exercise and following a low-cholesterol diet — it may be helpful in controlling cholesterol levels. Flaxseed may also be helpful for managing diabetes, relieving some menopausal symptoms and lowering the risk of heart disease. However, more research needs to be conducted to confirm these findings.

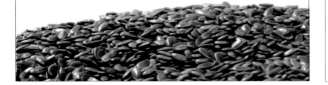

What the research says

Cancer
While some studies suggest that flaxseed may help reduce the formation and spread of certain cancers, more research needs to done to confirm these findings.

Heart (cardiovascular) disease
Some studies suggest that alpha-linolenic acid, which is found in flaxseed and flaxseed oil, may benefit people with heart disease. Early research also suggests that flaxseed may help lower high blood pressure, a condition that increases the risk of heart disease. However, more research is needed to determine whether flaxseed is effective for cardiovascular conditions.

Cholesterol levels
While flaxseed's effect on cholesterol seems promising, the research is mixed. Several studies show that taking between 3 and 50 grams of flaxseed a day can reduce total cholesterol and low-density lipoprotein (LDL), or "bad," cholesterol levels. In fact, some studies suggest that supplementing your diet with flaxseed may reduce total blood cholesterol by as much as 15 percent, and LDL cholesterol by as much as 18 percent. However, other studies aren't as favorable. For instance, in one study of postmenopausal women, flaxseed did not seem to have an effect on LDL cholesterol levels. More research is needed.

Diabetes
Research suggests that taking flaxseed may lower blood sugar levels in people with type 2 diabetes. However, the same results have not been found for flaxseed oil.

Menopausal symptoms
Women frequently use flaxseed to manage menopausal symptoms. Results have been mixed when it comes to flaxseed and the treatment of menopausal symptoms. While some evidence suggests that flaxseed may reduce symptoms such as hot flashes and night sweats, other studies have found no improvement.

Valerian

Valerian (*Valeriana officinalis*) is a tall, flowering grassland plant native to Europe and Asia. It is also found in North America. The roots and underground stems (rhizomes) of valerian are used to make teas and supplements, including capsules, tablets and liquid extracts.

Valerian has been used to treat insomnia for thousands of years — since the time of ancient Greece and Rome. Historically, valerian was used to treat nervousness, trembling, headaches and heart palpitations.

Today, this herb continues to be used for insomnia and anxiety-related sleep disorders, along with depression and anxiety, headaches, trembling disorders, attention-deficit/hyperactivity disorder (ADHD), and chronic fatigue syndrome. Valerian is also used for menstrual cramps and menopausal symptoms, including hot flashes.

Valerian is generally considered safe to use for short periods of time. Side effects, which are typically mild, may include headaches, dizziness, upset stomach and morning fatigue after taking a dose. Because its safety during long-term use is unknown, don't take valerian for more than four to six weeks at a time. Also, be cautious about drinking alcohol while taking valerian, as the combination may have a sedative effect.

Our take

Valerian appears to be beneficial for insomnia — and may have positive effects on anxiety, menstrual cramps and menopausal symptoms. However, further research is necessary to draw definitive conclusions.

Because valerian is generally safe at recommended doses, it may be worthwhile to try this supplement if you face these conditions. Just don't take valerian for more than four to six weeks at a time, as long-term safety is not known.

Finally, one more tip: If you'd like to try valerian to treat your insomnia, take the supplement an hour or two before bedtime. That's when results have been best.

What the research says

Here's what some of the research suggests:

Anxiety
There is contradictory evidence about the effectiveness of valerian for anxiety. In some studies, people who used valerian reported less anxiety and stress. In other studies, people reported no benefit.

Insomnia
Much of the available research suggests that valerian can help you fall asleep and may improve sleep quality. In fact, in a review of 18 clinical trials on valerian's effect on insomnia, researchers found that valerian increased the chance of improved sleep quality. However, other studies have not found significant improvements in insomnia when compared to an inactive substance (placebo). More research is needed to determine exactly what role valerian might play in sleep.

Menstrual pain and menopausal symptoms
Early research suggests that valerian may reduce the duration of menstrual pain, including cramps. And in one study on postmenopausal women, researchers found that valerian did reduce menopausal symptoms, including the number of hot flashes. However, much more research needs to be conducted to confirm these findings.

Other uses
There is not enough scientific evidence to determine whether valerian works for other conditions, such as depression and stress. Researchers continue to study other potential uses for valerian.

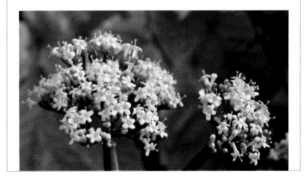

Ginger

Ginger (*Zingiber officinale*) is a plant with leafy stems and greenish-purple flowers that is native to Asia. The plant's underground stem (rhizome) produces an aromatic spice that is often used in Asian cooking.

Ginger supplements are made from this underground stem. Ginger is available as a powder, tablet, extract, tincture and oil.

Traditionally, ginger has been used to relieve nausea from pregnancy (morning sickness), as well as nausea related to motion sickness, chemotherapy and use of anesthesia during surgery. Ginger may also be used to treat pain associated with menstrual cramps and arthritis.

Ginger is considered safe when taken in small doses. Side effects, which are typically mild, may include gas, bloating and heartburn — especially when taking ginger in powder form. Ginger is not recommended for nausea during pregnancy if you have a history of bleeding disorders or miscarriages.

Our take

Ginger gets a green light because it's been shown to be somewhat effective in reducing morning sickness and in delaying motion sickness and speeding recovery from it. It's also shown promise for treating painful menstrual cramps.

Ginger is generally considered safe when taken in small amounts and for a short time. High doses can cause abdominal discomfort.

Before taking ginger to prevent nausea associated with pregnancy, talk with your health care provider. And avoid ginger if you take anticoagulant medications, because it may increase bleeding risk.

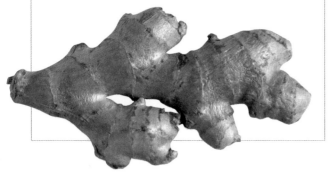

What the research says

Here's what some studies have found:

Arthritis
When it comes to ginger's effectiveness in treating osteoarthritis, rheumatoid arthritis, and joint or muscle pain, results are mixed. Some research suggests that ginger may modestly improve the pain associated with osteoarthritis. However, many of these studies have been small. And there hasn't been enough evidence to determine if ginger can play a role in improving rheumatoid arthritis. More research is needed.

Dysmenorrhea
Research shows that ginger can reduce pain in women with painful menstrual cramps (dysmenorrhea). In one analysis of related studies, taking ginger powder during the first three to four days of a menstrual cycle decreased pain in women with dysmenorrhea by up to 85 percent compared with an inactive ingredient (placebo).

Nausea
Results are mixed when it comes to using ginger for nausea. Perhaps the most promising results have come from ginger's effect on pregnancy-related nausea. Studies suggest that ginger may help ease nausea from pregnancy when used for short periods. However, it can take a few days for ginger to work.

Results on the effectiveness of ginger to prevent or relieve nausea from chemotherapy and anesthesia have been inconsistent. Some studies have found ginger to reduce nausea in these instances. In one study, for instance, researchers found that taking ginger before surgery significantly reduced the incidence of nausea after surgery. And a few trials have found that ginger helped control nausea after chemotherapy. However, other studies have had less positive results.

And when it comes to ginger and motion sickness, the research just isn't there. Most evidence suggests that ginger doesn't prevent motion sickness. More research is needed.

Supplements for lipids

Lipids are the fats found in your blood. The most well-known lipid is cholesterol, but there are other kinds, too. Your body needs lipids to work properly, but an excess of lipids can increase your risk of heart disease. You can reduce your lipid levels by eating a healthy, low-fat diet, exercising regularly and reaching a healthy weight. Medications are often recommended, as well.

Research has found that some dietary supplements may help maintain or lower lipid levels in your blood. Two of these supplements are plant sterols and red yeast rice.

Plant sterols

Plant sterols help block the absorption of cholesterol. They occur naturally in some oils, nuts and fruits. They are also added to some foods, including margarines, orange juices and yogurt drinks. Plant sterols are available as supplements, in tablets and capsules.

Our take

Consuming supplements and foods enriched with plant sterols is considered safe and can help reduce total blood cholesterol and low-density lipoprotein (LDL), or "bad," cholesterol levels. It's believed that 2 to 3 grams of plant sterols a day provides benefits.

What the research says

Research shows that plant sterols can help reduce total blood cholesterol and LDL cholesterol by as much as 15 percent. There is some evidence that results may be greater for those with high LDL cholesterol levels as opposed to those with normal or borderline levels.

Red yeast rice

Red yeast rice (*Monascus purpureus*) is the product of yeast grown on white rice. The powdered yeast-rice mixture is a dietary staple in Asia and has been used in traditional Chinese medicine.

Red yeast rice contains several compounds that appear to lower cholesterol levels. One of them is monacolin K, the same ingredient found in the prescription cholesterol-lowering drug lovastatin (Altoprev).

Don't take red yeast rice if you're already taking cholesterol medication. You also shouldn't use this supplement if you're pregnant or nursing. Use red yeast rice under the supervision of your doctor or other members of your health care team.

Our take

Red yeast rice is capable of lowering blood cholesterol levels. While the supplement is generally considered safe, it also carries the same potential side effects as statin cholesterol drugs.

The only advantage of taking red yeast rice in place of a statin drug may be the cheaper cost. However, with a supplement, there's less assurance regarding quality and how much active ingredient is actually in the product you buy. Some red yeast rice products may actually contain only small amounts of monacolin K, and thus have little effect on cholesterol levels.

What the research says

A number of studies indicate that red yeast rice containing considerable amounts of monacolin K can lower your total blood cholesterol level, your low-density lipoprotein (LDL), or "bad," cholesterol level and your triglyceride level.

Multivitamins: Do you need one?

The best way to get your vitamins and minerals is through a balanced diet. However, there are times when a supplement containing a variety of vitamins and minerals — commonly referred to as a multivitamin pill — may be appropriate.

If you don't get the recommended servings of fruits, vegetables and other healthy foods, you may benefit from a vitamin and mineral supplement. In addition, if you have to limit your diet because of food allergies or intolerance to certain foods, a supplement may be appropriate. Multivitamins are also recommended for strict vegetarians who eat no animal products. These individuals may not get enough vitamin B-12, zinc, iron and calcium.

If you're over age 65, there are a variety of reasons why you may not get the nutrients you need. A multivitamin may make more sense than taking single-nutrient pills.

It's generally recommended that women who are pregnant or breast-feeding take additional vitamins. Discuss what to take with your doctor.

What to watch for

Consider these points when choosing a multivitamin:

Iron. Although supplemental iron is advised during pregnancy and for iron deficiency anemia, too much iron can be toxic. For men and postmenopausal women, it's probably wise to take a pill with little or no iron — 8 milligrams (mg) a day or less. "Senior formulas" generally have less iron.

Vitamin B-6 (pyridoxine). Adequate levels of this vitamin may help lower blood homocysteine, a possible risk factor for heart attack, and improve immune system function. Older adults who lack variety in their diets may not get enough vitamin B-6, so a multivitamin that contains about 2 mg is often a good idea. Avoid excessive doses. Too much vitamin B-6 can result in nerve damage to the arms and legs, which is usually reversible when supplementation is stopped.

Vitamin B-12. Adequate levels of this vitamin may reduce your risk of anemia and age-related macular degeneration. Older adults often don't absorb this vitamin well. A multivitamin with at least 2 micrograms (mcg) may help.

Vitamin D. This vitamin helps the body absorb calcium and is essential in maintaining bone strength and bone density. Many older adults don't get regular exposure to sunlight and have trouble absorbing vitamin D, so taking a multivitamin with 600 to 800 international units (IU) will likely help improve bone health.

Vitamin E. A recent review of studies indicates that taking daily vitamin E supplements of 400 IU or more — and possibly as low as 150 IU — may pose health risks. Talk with your doctor before taking vitamin E supplements.

5 things to keep in mind

1. *Multivitamins don't need to cost much.* Most generic products and store brands are fine.
2. *Look for a third-party verification on the label, such as USP or NSF.* This means the product has been tested in a laboratory and meets standards of quality. (Learn more on page 200.)
3. *Look for a multivitamin that contains a wide variety of vitamins and minerals in the appropriate amounts.* Usually, you'll look for 100 percent of the Daily Value (DV). Check the contents to make sure you're not getting too much of any nutrient, which can be harmful. In most cases, if the tablet doesn't exceed 100 percent of the DV, it's considered safe.
4. *Take your multivitamin with food.* If it contains iron, don't take a calcium supplement at the same time, since iron interferes with calcium absorption.
5. *Be wary of claims such as "stress formula," "high potency," "natural" or "slow release."* They're often just marketing ploys and only add to the price.

Supplements to avoid

While certain herbal supplements are safe and even show promise in helping manage and even prevent certain conditions, other supplements are not safe and generally should be avoided.

Kava

Kava is a member of the pepper family whose root and underground stem, called the rhizome, are used in various forms to treat anxiety, insomnia and menopausal symptoms. Scientific studies provide some evidence that kava may help manage anxiety, but the Food and Drug Administration (FDA) has issued a warning that using kava supplements can cause severe liver damage, including hepatitis and liver failure, possibly leading to death. Kava may also interact unfavorably with several drugs, including drugs used for Parkinson's disease.

Ephedra

Another herbal supplement to beware of is ephedra, whose main active ingredient, ephedrine, is known to stimulate the nervous system and heart. Ephedra has been used as an ingredient in dietary supplements designed to help people lose weight, boost their energy and improve their athletic performance. These marketing claims made ephedra very attractive to a wide range of people, but the science doesn't support the hype.

Between 1995 and 1997, the FDA received more than 900 reports of possible ephedra toxicity. Serious adverse events such as stroke, heart attack and sudden death were reported in 37 cases. In 2001, a Minnesota Vikings lineman died after collapsing during one of the team's summer workouts. Then in 2003, Baltimore Orioles pitcher Steve Bechler died during spring training. Products containing ephedra were linked to both deaths.

In 2004, the FDA banned the sale of dietary supplements containing ephedra in the United States. But it's important to note that this ban doesn't apply to traditional Chinese herbal remedies or to products such as herbal teas regulated as conventional foods.

Bitter orange

Bitter orange is a tree whose oil is used in foods, cosmetics and aromatherapy products. After ephedra was banned, many herbal weight-loss products began using concentrated extracts of bitter orange peel instead of ephedra. But it's important to note that bitter orange contains the chemical synephrine, which is similar to the main chemical in ephedra. Presently, there's not a lot of evidence that bitter orange is any safer than ephedra, or that taking it will result in permanent weight loss.

Yohimbe

The bark of the yohimbe tree contains a chemical called yohimbine. As a dietary supplement, the dried bark of the yohimbe tree is made into tea and taken by mouth. An extract of the bark is also put into capsules and tablets.

Yohimbine lowers blood pressure and increases blood flow to the genitals. Traditionally, it's been used in Africa to increase sexual desire. Currently, it's used to treat sexual dysfunction, including erectile dysfunction in men.

A drug form of yohimbine — called yohimbine hydrochloride — has been studied for erectile dysfunction and is considered safe if taken under a doctor's supervision.

Yohimbe can cause severe side effects, including high blood pressure, a racing heartbeat, kidney failure, headache, anxiety, dizziness, nausea, vomiting, tremors and sleeplessness. The herb can be very dangerous if you take too much of it or take it over a long period of time. Finally, it's important to know that the amount of yohimbine in dietary supplements varies widely, and some products contain very little of the herb.

Spa: Rejuvenating mind, body and spirit

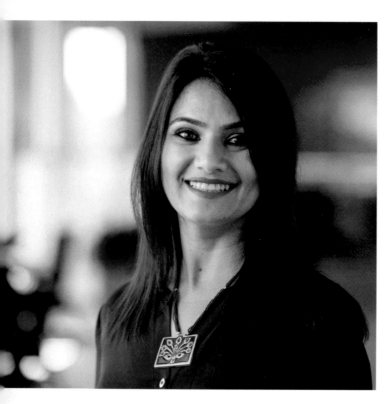

Anjali Bhagra, M.D.
Executive and International Medicine

Dr. Bhagra is education chair of Integrative Medicine and Health at Mayo Clinic in Rochester, Minnesota.

A visit with Dr. Bhagra

In this section, you'll learn about spa therapies and the unique ways they can improve how you feel — and enhance your wellness.

Spa therapies can be a helpful addition to your wellness routine for three reasons. First, there's nothing negative about going to a spa. You don't need a medical diagnosis to go to a spa, and you don't need someone to give you a prescription for a massage. The choice to go to a spa is entirely in your hands. This can be very empowering.

Second, as you'll learn in this section, most of the therapies offered at a spa are safe treatments that can enhance your wellness.

Finally, most spa therapies are relaxing and can boost your resilience. Resilience is your ability to bounce back from life's challenges. Resilience can be viewed in four different ways.

- Physical resilience: being strong and healthy enough to recover from illness or injury
- Emotional resilience: experiencing positive emotions and recovering quickly from negative ones
- Spiritual resilience: being able to maintain a higher meaning even in the face of disappointment and adversity
- Mental resilience: your ability to stay focused when you're faced with stress

As a Mayo Clinic physician, I try to help my patients in two very distinct ways: treatment and healing. Treatment is very specific. For example, I can give you an antibiotic to treat your pneumonia. But healing from that pneumonia is very different. After treatment has cured your pneumonia, you may still be dealing with its effects, such as chest pain and a cough. That's where integrative therapies — and in this case, spa therapies — can be healing.

You deserve to be able to make choices that help you feel good and improve your overall wellness. Added to your overall wellness routine, spa therapies offer an opportunity to do just that.

History of spas

When you hear the term *spa*, what images come to mind? Perhaps it elicits an image of pampering. Or maybe you've become accustomed to hearing the term spa used often, to describe everything from a nail spa to a dog spa.

What is a spa?

Although the term *spa* can mean many things to different people, the historical definition of spa is "a place that promotes health and healing."

At their core, spa services are evidence-based therapies designed to help promote health — therapies that can be a good fit in any ongoing personal wellness program. At their core, spas are places of rest, health, rejuvenation, relaxation and regeneration, achieved through some form of water. Spas are used all over the world; in the United States, the first spa was started in the 1850s in Saratoga Springs, New York.

While the popular use of the term *spa* may have changed over time, the connection between wellness and spa therapies has strengthened in recent years. The terms *wellness* and *spa* are even being used interchangeably when the goal of a spa experience is to help people maintain and improve health.

A shift in focus

As the spa industry continues to grow, spas are turning to a focus on wellness and integrative health as a way to distinguish themselves from the competition. This focus is gaining attention in the U.S., where some believe that spas will connect health care with disease prevention — or, in a broader sense, will connect traditional medicine and integrative medicine. A focus on relaxation and stress relief is a top priority for spas interested in following this trend.

To this day, spa therapy is often prescribed by doctors in Europe for the treatment of specific health issues, and studies confirm its benefits. And recent research also shows that spa therapies — in particular, various types of water-related therapy — are helpful in managing the symptoms of fibromyalgia. Spa therapies also are commonly prescribed in Europe to treat low back pain.

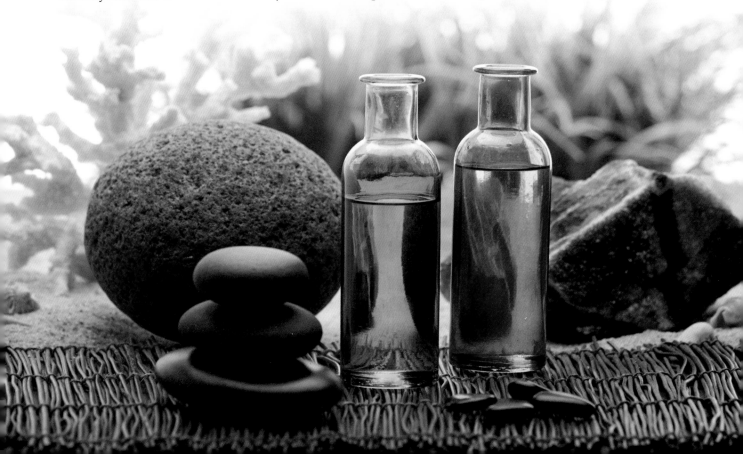

Spa and wellness

In earlier sections of this book, you learned about many things you can do for yourself to enhance your wellness. This is where spa therapies differ. A spa may be the one and only place where someone does something for you in terms of your wellness — whether you're getting a massage, a facial or another type of spa therapy. In a spa setting, a massage may offer a break in the midst of a hectic time in your life and help you refocus your energy on how you can improve your wellness. In addition, experiencing spa therapies may recharge your battery, so to speak, providing you with encouragement to take other steps that can improve your health, your wellness and your quality of life overall.

Although the term *spa* means different things to different people, spa therapies can aid in enhancing wellness through a variety of practices, some of which you've already read about in this book. You will read about others in this section.

- **Massage.** Massage is often offered at spas, both with and without aromatherapy. In addition to traditional styles of massage that don't involve water, water and even clay may be applied to the massage experience at a spa. (Learn about massage and aromatherapy starting on page 82.)

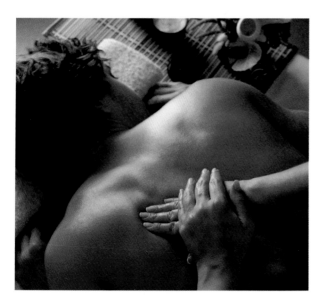

- **Relaxation therapies.** Many spas offer various types of relaxation therapies. Because wellness includes achieving a balance between body, mind and soul, some spas offer meditation classes and opportunities to help foster a sense of relaxation and nourishment of spirit. Spas offer an opportunity to try integrative practices such as these that you may then choose to use at home.
- **Aromatherapy.** Aromatherapy involves oils that evoke different feelings and sensations.
- **Acupuncture.** Many spas offer acupuncture to promote stress reduction and lessen pain. (Learn more starting on page 94.)
- **Saunas** (see page 130 in this section).
- **Hot tubs** (see page 132 in this section).
- **Skin care** (see page 135 in this section). Spas often offer a host of skin-related services, including facials and manicures. Receiving skin care services at a spa may give you an opportunity to see what other wellness-related services a spa offers. In turn, what may start as a skin care experience may serve as a gateway to other wellness practices that you may not have considered before.

As with any complementary treatment, it's important to remember that nothing is without risk. Some cosmetic treatments can be dangerous if not carried out properly. Protect yourself from bacteria by forgoing certain spa treatments if you have an open cut or wound.

When considering a spa, pay attention to how equipment is cleaned. Spa technicians generally should use new or sanitized instruments on your hands and feet. Technicians should use different files and clippers on each person.

In addition, be aware that health insurance does not cover most massage and other spa treatments, although some are covered by health savings accounts.

This section will introduce you to spa services, what they include and what current research says about their use. Here's a look at some of the services you may find in a spa and what's helpful to know about each one.

Saunas

Saunas have been used for hundreds of years, although they're known by different names across the world. Finnish people call them saunas. Native Americans call them sweat lodges. Russians call them banias. But no matter what they're called, they have one thing in common: They all offer the opportunity to feel better through heat and sweat.

Saunas can relax tense muscles and can cause reactions similar to what's experienced during moderate exercise: vigorous sweating and increased heart rate.

Use saunas in moderation and with caution, especially if you have uncontrolled diabetes or kidney disease, or have recently undergone gastric bypass surgery.

If you have a heart condition, research both supports and cautions against sauna use. Some research shows that saunas can pose risks to those with conditions such as unstable angina or those who have had a heart attack. On the other hand, research also shows that repeated sauna use can improve heart function.

As with all other integrative medicine practices, talk to your health care team about what is best for your personal situation.

Saunas at Mayo Clinic

Mayo Clinic has investigated the use of infrared saunas, which differ from traditional saunas because they use light to create heat. A traditional sauna uses heat to warm the air, which in turn warms your body. An infrared sauna heats your body directly without warming the air around you.

As with traditional saunas, infrared saunas can elicit a reaction in your body that's similar to that of moderate exercise. However, an infrared sauna produces these results at lower temperatures than does a traditional sauna. This can make an infrared sauna a good option for people who could benefit from the experience of a sauna but can't tolerate the heat of a conventional sauna. More research on infrared saunas is needed to confirm these benefits.

Our take

Several studies have looked at using infrared saunas to treat chronic health problems such as high blood pressure, congestive heart failure and rheumatoid arthritis and found some evidence of benefit. However, larger and more-rigorous studies are needed to confirm these results; most of these studies were small. Even so, if you're interested in exploring another option for relaxation, saunas can be a safe way to do so. Discuss sauna use with your health care team first to ensure that it's a safe option for you.

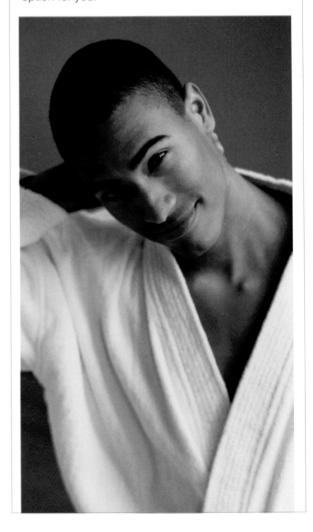

What the research says

Rheumatic conditions

Rheumatic disease includes a range of conditions, such as arthritis, lupus and fibromyalgia. For those with rheumatic conditions, researchers have found that saunas can help improve joint mobility and reduce pain. In one small study in particular, people with rheumatoid arthritis who took part in infrared and far-infrared sauna therapy twice a week for four weeks had significantly less stiffness.

Attention-deficit/hyperactivity disorder (ADHD)

Some research shows that saunas can be helpful for people who have ADHD and related disorders.

Asthma and bronchitis

Researchers have found that saunas can help improve breathing in people with asthma and bronchitis. Note that it's best not to use a sauna while in the midst of a respiratory infection.

Chronic obstructive pulmonary disease (COPD)

Researchers who conducted a small study of 12 men from the Netherlands found that regular sauna therapy improved lung function.

Common cold

Research shows that people who visited a sauna twice a week for six months were half as likely to catch the common cold.

Heart disease

Saunas may help treat various forms of heart disease. Infrared and far-infrared saunas, for example, seem to benefit blood pressure levels.

Chronic pain

Researchers who studied 46 people hospitalized for chronic pain found that those who had infrared or far-infrared sauna treatment five days a week for four weeks showed fewer signs of pain. Two years later, most who previously had sauna treatment could return to work.

Depression

In a study of 28 people with mild depression, those who took part in 20 infrared and far-infrared sauna sessions over four weeks had fewer symptoms of depression, had more of an appetite and were more able to relax.

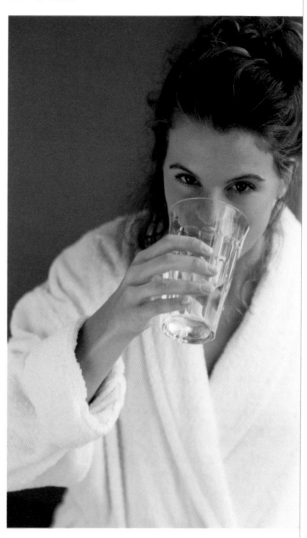

Hot tubs and warm pools

Hot tubs are another common spa experience. You can find hot tubs at pools, spas and hotels. Hot water can relax tight muscles and ease tension.

At one point, hot tubs and warm pools caused concern for safety in people, so Mayo Clinic researchers studied 15 men with stable coronary artery disease and found no problems in a typical 15-minute soak in 104-degree water.

They found that soaking in a hot tub offers benefits similar to those from exercise, with less stress on the heart. Soaking in a hot tub increases your heart rate while lowering your blood pressure.

However, hot tubs aren't for everyone. Don't use a hot tub if you have any sort of wound, have severe respiratory problems or are pregnant.

In addition, hot tubs can be a breeding ground for dozens of types of bacteria, many of them potential pathogens. The water also can be ground zero for infectious diseases. In one study that tested 43 water samples from whirlpool bathtubs — both private and public — researchers found that all 43 had bacterial growth ranging from mild to dangerous. Bacteria found in hot tubs can lead to numerous diseases, such as urinary tract infections, septicemia, pneumonia and several types of skin infections.

Another potential complication of using a hot tub is a condition Mayo Clinic diagnosed called hot tub lung. This condition causes coughing, shortness of breath and fever, all from bacteria inhaled from a hot tub.

Although hot tubs can offer benefits, these are all good reasons to approach hot tubs with caution. For some, a calm warm pool or a hot bath is a better option. Warm water helps by stimulating blood flow to stiff muscles and frozen joints, which can aid in gentle stretching that promotes flexibility.

Our take

As with any therapy, hot tub therapy can have both positive and negative effects. If you're interested in trying a hot tub, talk with your doctor first to make sure that it's safe for you. If it is, and you enjoy it, you may have found another piece of your wellness routine.

What the research says

Studies show that warm water can be beneficial in helping manage conditions that involve pain. Here's what researchers have discovered.

Arthritis and fibromyalgia
Arthritis experts promote the use of warm-water pools as a way to reduce the force of gravity that's compressing a joint, support sore limbs, decrease swelling and inflammation, and increase circulation — all in just 20 minutes. Warm water can be helpful in reducing the pain and stiffness of arthritis. A variety of studies show that people who have arthritis and take part in a warm-water exercise program two or three times a week often are able to move more easily and experience significantly less pain. These exercise programs provided an emotional boost, helped people sleep better and were particularly effective for people who were overweight.

Fibromyalgia
As with arthritis, researchers have found that warm water can help ease pain associated with fibromyalgia. In one study, researchers followed 33 women for 12 weeks and found that warm-water pool-based exercise, done twice a week for 12 weeks, helped decrease their pain. In fact, older women and those who had more intense pain showed the most improvement.

Expert insight

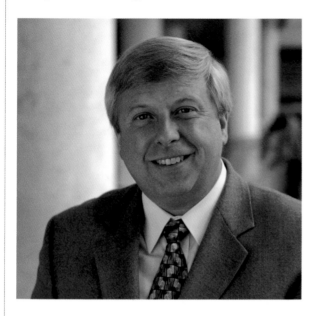

Brent A. Bauer, M.D.

Medical editor, *Mayo Clinic Guide to Integrative Medicine*

In addition to his role as a medical editor of this book, Dr. Bauer is involved in many areas of the Mayo Clinic practice. He is director of research in Integrative Medicine and Health, as well as medical director of Rejuvenate Spa at the Mayo Clinic Healthy Living Program at Mayo Clinic in Rochester, Minnesota.

Why does Mayo Clinic have a spa?

It's not news that people are looking for effective ways to prevent disease and promote health — while still treating disease. Integrative medicine is a huge part of this push. That's why wellness programs, healthy living classes, and spa services — all of which can improve well-being — are featured at the Mayo Clinic Healthy Living Program in Rochester, Minnesota.

Why spa services, in particular?

Rejuvenate Spa opened at Mayo Clinic in 2014 and offers an array of integrative therapies, including body massage and aesthetic treatments such as facials and body wraps, manicure, pedicure, and waxing services. The setting itself is designed to be a tranquil environment that embodies the essence of wellness, a key element in the traditional idea of what a spa is.

How does this differ from other types of spas?

Not all "spas" you hear of are designed exactly for this purpose. In today's world, you may hear of many different types of "spas" — nail spas, dog spas, and so on.

But when I think of what a spa truly is, I think of more traditional descriptions. In that sense, spas are places where you "take the waters," or in Europe, "take a cure." A spa can be an evidence-based practice that provides activities and therapies designed to enhance your overall personal wellness. Mayo Clinic opened Rejuvenate Spa for this very reason.

Did medical research, such as the findings in this book, play a role in Mayo Clinic's decision to open a spa?

Mayo Clinic is an academic medical center, so it may not come as a surprise that 15 years of research at Mayo Clinic led to the opening of a spa on the institution's Rochester, Minnesota, campus.

The findings — similar to what you're reading about in this book — were overwhelming. For example, we learned that therapies such as massage not only make people feel better but also reduce stress levels, improve mood and help treat common medical issues, such as low back pain. In short, we discovered that spa therapies have a lot to offer anyone visiting Mayo Clinic.

Making services such as massage and acupuncture available in a spa setting is a way to make these wellness-enhancing treatments available to more people. This is especially important for patients and families who travel to Rochester for care and could benefit from an opportunity to relieve stress and pain, as well as improve quality of life overall.

Learn more about Rejuvenate Spa at the Mayo Clinic Healthy Living Program at *https://healthyliving. mayoclinic.org/services-/rejuvenate-spa.php.*

Finding a spa in your community

A true, comprehensive spa can provide elements of wellness that can help you achieve your health and wellness goals. If you're ready to take the first step, you may wonder: *How can I find a spa that fits my needs and preferences?*

Rejuvenate Spa at Mayo Clinic's Healthy Living Center may help provide an example of what to look for. Although Rejuvenate Spa is more of a destination spa than may be appropriate for everyday wellness, it offers some tips on what to look for when you're researching spas in your community.

Rejuvenate Spa offers many spa services, including massage, facials and body treatments. At the same time, Rejuvenate Spa is not a stand-alone spa — it's located within the Mayo Clinic Healthy Living Program at Mayo Clinic's Dan Abraham Healthy Living Center, which offers wellness classes focused on nutrition, physical activity, relaxation, stress management and resiliency, and meditation, as well as one-on-one health coaching. The focus of Rejuvenate Spa brings together everything addressed in this book: stress management through massage or meditation training, aromatherapy and yoga, as well as exercise opportunities and healthy eating.

If you don't have a comprehensive wellness center in your community that offers all of the same tenets of wellness as the Mayo Clinic Healthy Living Program, look for a place that can teach you self-care skills and that also offers massage or a healthy-living class. Depending on your location, you may need to put your program together a la carte.

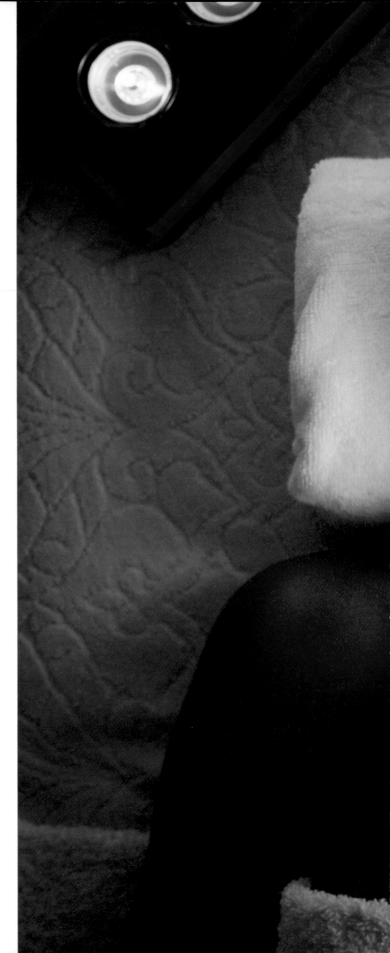

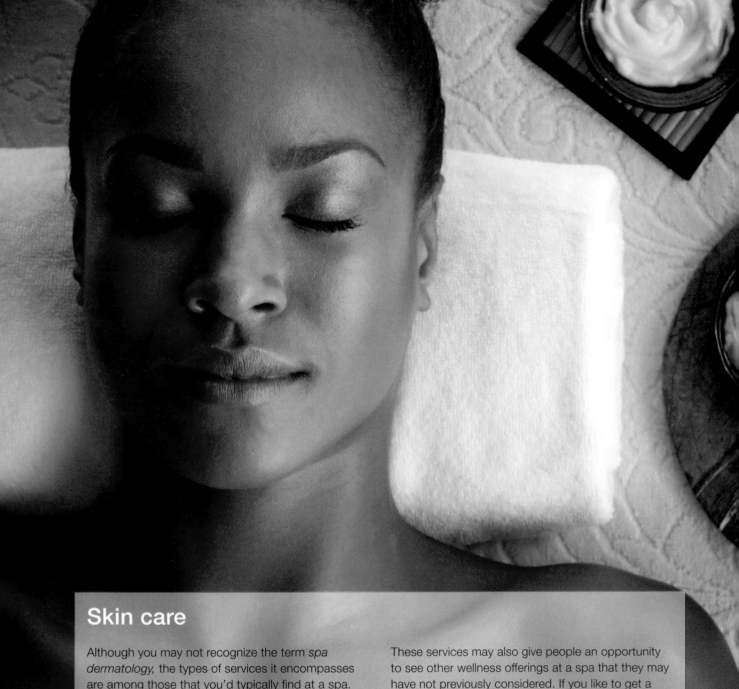

Skin care

Although you may not recognize the term *spa dermatology,* the types of services it encompasses are among those that you'd typically find at a spa.

Skin care services at a spa include microdermabrasion, laser treatments, Botox treatments, manicures and pedicures. Spa services such as these can turn into the first step in a wellness journey for people, simply because the services help people feel better about themselves.

These services may also give people an opportunity to see other wellness offerings at a spa that they may have not previously considered. If you like to get a manicure or pedicure, find a reputable spa that uses clean techniques and enjoy the experience. While you are there, ask about other services or therapies that might enhance your wellness. The pedicure or manicure that you're used to enjoying may lead you down a new path that can ultimately improve your overall well-being.

Other approaches

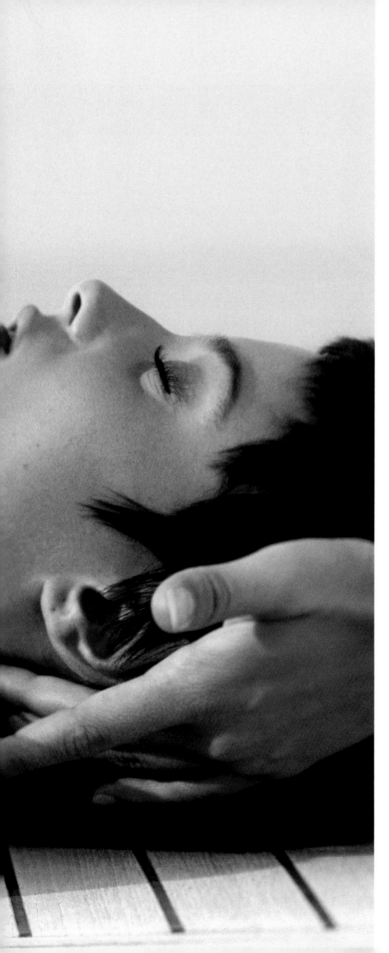

This section takes a look at all-encompassing approaches to health and healing. Here you will find information about complete medical systems that are quite different from traditional Western medicine. You may hear these systems referred to as "whole medical systems" because they are used to explain, diagnose and treat diseases.

This type of medicine is practiced by individual cultures and is largely based on traditional customs, many of which date back thousands of years and originate from a variety of cultures.

These all-encompassing approaches to health and healing are based on the beliefs that there is a powerful connection between mind and body and that the body has the power to heal itself. Treatments that comprise the integrative medical systems that you'll read about focus on prevention and on achieving a healthy "balance." They promote diet, exercise, sleep and daily routines to maintain wellness and encourage healing.

One of the differing points between integrative medical systems and conventional medicine is that treatments are individualized. No two individuals with similar symptoms receive the exact same treatment. For example, two women who undergo menopause and experience hot flashes may see the same traditional Chinese medicine practitioner. However, they may receive different forms of acupuncture therapy and different herbs, depending on their individual diagnoses.

To date, research has generally focused only on studying individual components of these medical systems and not the whole system, which is more complex. For example, there's research supporting the use of acupuncture in the management of pain, as well as nausea and vomiting. But acupuncture is only one component of traditional Chinese medicine.

Research on the effectiveness of whole medical systems is ongoing, and results are eagerly awaited. For now, read about the latest research findings and get general information about these approaches to integrative medicine.

Ayurveda

Ayurveda, which means "science of life," originated in India thousands of years ago and is thought to be one of the world's oldest systems of medical practices.

The basic theories on which ayurvedic medicine is based are that all things in the universe are joined together and that all forms of life consist of combinations of three energy elements: wind, fire and water. When these elements are balanced, a person is healthy. When they're unbalanced, the body is weakened and susceptible to illness.

To restore harmony and balance and treat illness, some of the therapies used by ayurvedic practitioners include:

- Enemas, fasting, or use of certain foods or metals to eliminate impurities and cleanse the body
- Breathing exercises, herbs or certain foods to reduce symptoms
- Massage of the body's "vital points," where life energy is stored, to reduce pain and fatigue or improve circulation
- Therapies such as yoga and meditation to reduce worry and anxiety and promote balance and harmony

In India, ayurvedic medicine is still practiced by the majority of the population, although it exists side by side with conventional Western medicine. According to the 2012 National Health Interview Survey, almost 250,000 U.S. adults used ayurvedic medicine in the previous year.

Body elements

Ayurvedic medicine is based on specific beliefs as to how the body functions.

Prana

An important concept of ayurvedic medicine is that the human body houses a vital life energy called *prana*. Prana — similar to *qi* in traditional Chinese medicine and *ki* in traditional Japanese medicine — is the basis of life and healing.

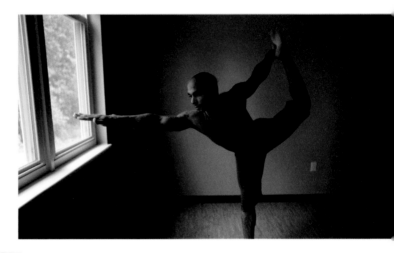

Doshas

As this vital life energy circulates throughout the body, it's influenced by elements called *doshas*. Doshas control the basic activities of the body and formulate important individual characteristics. The ayurvedic belief is that a balance of doshas is necessary for optimal health.

Each dosha is composed of a combination of basic elements: space (ether), air, fire, water and earth. These elements represent subtle qualities of life energy and how the energy expresses itself within the body.

Doshas are influenced by diet, activity and body processes and are continuously being formulated and reformulated.

An imbalance in a particular dosha will produce symptoms related to that dosha, which are different from symptoms produced by an imbalance in another dosha.

Prakriti

Certain doshas are predominant in each individual and determine that person's "constitution." The ayurvedic term for constitution is *prakriti*.

Your constitution refers to your general health, how likely your body is to become out of balance, and your body's ability to resist or recover from illness. Ayurvedic belief is that your constitution does not change over your lifetime.

Details on doshas

Each dosha has essential physical and psychological characteristics.
- **Vata dosha.** The vata dosha controls movement and essential body processes such as cell division, the heart, breathing and the mind. It can be thrown off balance by staying up late.
- **Pitta dosha.** The pitta dosha is believed to control the body's hormones and digestive system. When it's out of balance, a person may experience negative emotions or digestive symptoms.
- **Kapha dosha.** The kapha dosha is thought to help maintain strength and immunity and control growth. People with kapha as their main dosha are thought to be vulnerable to diabetes, cancer, obesity and respiratory illnesses.

Our take

Some treatments used in ayurvedic medicine, such as yoga, massage or meditation, appear to be safe and may be effective.

There's likely little risk in giving ayurveda a try. However, good-quality scientific studies on ayurvedic practices are limited. Many therapies — especially those involving herbs or metals — don't have enough scientific data to recommend their use.

In addition, ayurvedic medications sometimes can be toxic to the body. Many materials used in them haven't been studied thoroughly, so make sure to talk to your health care team before trying an ayurvedic supplement and use it only under your doctor's close supervision.

What the research says

Cardiovascular disease
Targeting several aspects of heart disease, researchers have learned that:
- The herbal and mineral formulation *abana* may reduce the frequency and severity of angina pain.
- A bark powder called *terminalia arjuna* may help chest pain following a heart attack, and seems to be helpful in treating congestive heart failure.
- The traditional ayurvedic herbal remedy MAK-4 may be useful in preventing the effects of low-density lipoprotein (LDL), also known as "bad" cholesterol, that contributes to heart disease.

Cognitive function
The herb *brahmi* may improve memory and cognitive function.

Diabetes
Although a range of herbs and herbal formulations have been said to help manage and even prevent diabetes, studies using ayurvedic remedies have produced mixed results.

Neurodegenerative diseases
Although more study is needed, ashwagandha — roots of *Withania somnifera* — may be helpful in treating Alzheimer's disease and spinal cord injury, as well as Parkinson's disease and Huntington's disease.

Vitiligo
Root powder from the herb *Picrorhiza kurroa* may help treat the skin condition vitiligo.

Obesity
Some research shows that the ayurvedic herb *guggul* (Medohar) may contribute to weight loss, but more research is needed to confirm these findings.

Arthritis
Certain herbal ayurvedic formulations seem to be effective in helping treat osteoarthritis, especially osteoarthritis of the knees. There is also evidence that a formula called RA-11 and *Curcuma longa* (turmeric) may reduce joint swelling in rheumatoid arthritis, but other research showed no benefit.

Naturopathy

Naturopathy is a form of health care based on the belief that the body has an innate healing power that can establish, maintain and restore health when it's in a healthy environment.

In naturopathy, the emphasis is on supporting health rather than combating disease. As such, naturopathic medicine relies on natural remedies, such as sunlight, air and water, along with "natural" supplements to promote well-being.

Early naturopaths often prescribed hydrotherapy — soaks in hot springs and other water-related therapies — to promote health. Today, naturopathic practitioners draw on many forms of integrative medicine, including practices such as massage, acupuncture, stress reduction, herbal remedies, practitioner-guided detoxification, exercise and lifestyle counseling.

Practitioners of naturopathy believe that health and healing should come in the most gentle, least invasive and most efficient manner possible.

Individuals who provide naturopathic care aren't all the same. A *naturopath* is a therapist who practices naturopathy. A *naturopathic physician* is a primary health care provider trained in a broad scope of naturopathic practices in addition to a standard medical curriculum. Both use the designation of N.D. — representing either naturopathic diploma or naturopathic doctor — which can cause confusion about the person's scope of practice, education and training.

Our take

If you are trying to stay healthy and well, a naturopathic physician may be a great partner to help guide you to healthy foods, exercise and other wellness practices. They can also offer guidance for many minor ailments and illnesses. But in cases of a serious medical condition, such as a heart attack or cancer, it's best to turn to modern medicine. Naturopathy may offer more in terms of wellness promotion, but your conventional health care team is best when it comes to treating and managing medical conditions when something more than self-care is needed.

What the research says

There haven't been any quality research studies conducted on naturopathy as a whole — a complete system of medicine. There's no evidence that naturopathic medicine can cure cancer or any other disease.

A limited number of studies have been done on herbs used as naturopathic treatments. For example, some research shows that echinacea can help prevent and treat the common cold, but some of the research that's been done isn't of good enough quality, which makes their findings less useful. Other research has been done on echinacea in terms of treating anxiety, treating gingivitis, improving how well the flu vaccine works and boosting exercise performance, but to date, the research that's been done isn't strong enough to show how well it works either way.

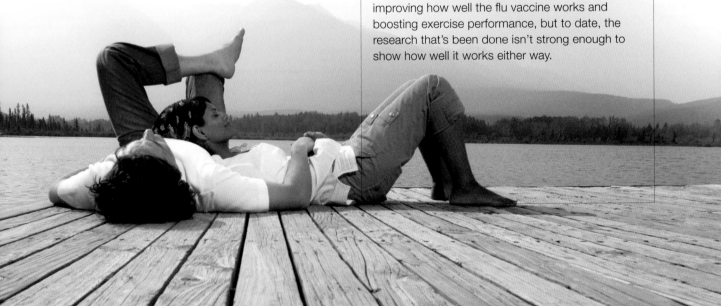

Traditional Chinese medicine

Traditional Chinese medicine is based on the belief that the body is a delicate balance of two complementary yet opposing forces: yin and yang. Health is achieved by maintaining an appropriate balance of the two.

An imbalance of yin and yang leads to blockage in the flow of blood and vital life energy (*qi*). To help unblock these pathways and restore health, practitioners of traditional Chinese medicine generally use one or a combination of treatments, which may include acupuncture, moxibustion or cupping; Chinese herbs; and massage and manipulation.

Moxibustion involves applying heat from burning of the herb moxa at an acupuncture point. Cupping involves placing a heated cup over a part of the body. As the air inside cools, its volume decreases, creating a slight suction and stimulating blood flow.

Chinese herbs are usually processed as teas, capsules, liquid extracts, granules or powders — but the raw, dried forms common centuries ago are still used. In all, there are more than 2,000 Chinese herbs.

Our take

In China, more than half of the population still uses traditional Chinese herbal preparations. Traditional Chinese medicine is integrated into the country's health care system and used side by side with modern medicine. In the United States, use of traditional Chinese medicine is growing; people generally pick and choose certain components of traditional Chinese medicine and use them in isolation. Practices such as acupuncture, massage and manipulation can be of benefit in treating certain conditions. A few Chinese herbs may also be of use in treating conditions such as cardiovascular disease and side effects of cancer. However, Chinese herbs need to be approached with caution. They can be very powerful, and some are dangerous. Ephedra (ma huang), the main active ingredient in many "natural" weight-loss products, is thought to have caused 22 deaths and 800 cases of toxicity.

What the research says

The individual component within traditional Chinese medicine that has received the most study is acupuncture. Only a few good studies have been conducted on Chinese herbs. That's because most Chinese herbs are used in combination, not alone, which makes them more difficult to study.

Autoimmune and inflammatory disease
The Chinese herb thunder god vine appears to relieve symptoms of rheumatoid arthritis, including pain, as well as tender and swollen joints. It also seems to improve physical function. Researchers have found that taking this herb with nonsteroidal anti-inflammatory medication adds to symptom relief. However, it may affect your immune system and cause decreased bone mineral density.

Cancer
Studies suggest Chinese herbs may shrink tumors, reduce side effects and improve response to treatment. But the quality of the studies has been weak.

Cardiovascular disease
Chinese herb formulas are taken to reduce symptoms of angina, stabilize abnormal heart rhythms, and improve heart function and blood composition. While there's some evidence of potential benefits, the studies have been limited and of poor design.

Knee osteoarthritis
A recent study shows the Chinese therapy tai chi can effectively treat symptoms of knee arthritis in older adults as well as standard physical therapy could.

Acupressure

Acupressure is based on the same ideas as acupuncture. But instead of inserting a needle, the practitioner applies physical pressure to specific points on the surface of the body using a finger, hand, elbow or device. The intent is to restore the flow of life energy, or *qi*.

Some people use acupressure simply as a relaxation technique, but it's also used to treat a variety of conditions, including musculoskeletal pain and tension, depression, anxiety, sleep difficulties, headaches, and nausea.

Numerous scientific studies support the use of acupressure applied to a specific point on the wrist known as P6 to prevent and treat nausea associated with chemotherapy and surgery, as well as nausea related to the morning sickness that may accompany pregnancy. Some people have found that wrist acupressure also helps reduce motion sickness. The P6 point is located about three finger-widths from the large crease in your wrist.

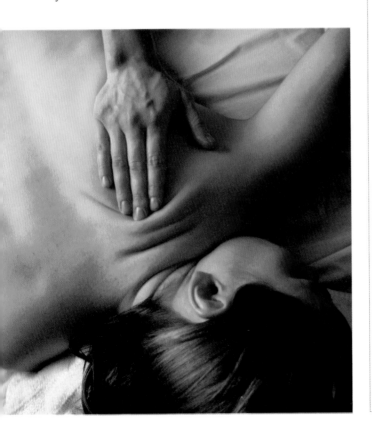

Our take

Using an acupressure band with a button that stimulates the P6 point on your wrist is a reasonable self-care strategy to try if you're interested in acupressure.

What the research says

Although more study is needed, research shows that acupressure may help treat these conditions:

Back pain
When compared with physical therapy, acupressure significantly lessened pain and disability in people with chronic low back pain, according to researchers. Other research shows that adding acupressure massage and aromatherapy to conventional treatment reduces pain and helps improve how well people with low back pain can walk.

Nausea and vomiting
A study of 20 trials shows that acupressure can lessen nausea and vomiting following surgery, but other research showed that it did not help reduce these symptoms. In terms of nausea related to morning sickness, acupressure wristbands haven't been found to be more effective than sham therapies, but some women find them helpful.

Eczema
Of several types of integrative medicine studied in helping treat eczema (atopic dermatitis), one study showed that four weeks of acupressure led to fewer itching and scaling symptoms.

Menstrual cramps
Although research on acupressure and menstrual cramps is limited, it appears that acupressure may be more effective than a placebo in easing menstrual cramps.

Reflexology

The theory behind reflexology is that specific areas on the soles of your feet correspond to other parts of your body — such as your head or neck or your internal organs.

Reflexologists use foot charts to guide them as they massage, and then apply varying amounts of manual pressure to specific areas of the feet in an effort to influence a problem elsewhere in the body. Sometimes, reflexologists also use items such as rubber balls, rubber bands or sticks of wood to assist in their work. The practice was developed by William Fitzgerald, M.D., in the early 20th century.

Reflexology is practiced primarily as a form of treatment for a variety of problems. However, some reflexologists also claim to diagnose certain illnesses based on the condition of the soles of a person's feet.

Reflexology is sometimes combined with other hands-on therapies, and may be offered by chiropractors and physical therapists.

What the research says

Although some research has been done on reflexology, more research is needed. Here are the most current research findings, all of which require further research.

Anxiety
There is preliminary evidence that reflexology may be helpful in aiding in relaxation.

Menopause symptoms
Preliminary research suggests reflexology may reduce some symptoms of menopause, but the reduction wasn't significant.

Pain
Some research has shown that reflexology may reduce the pain of migraines and other headaches, as well as cancer-related pain; however, the reduction in pain lasted only a short time.

Our take

There's little risk involved in reflexology, and massaging the soles of your feet can feel good. But there's also not much evidence to indicate that the therapy can treat various diseases or symptoms, as its practitioners claim. Among most conventional doctors, the theory behind reflexology is a little difficult to grasp.

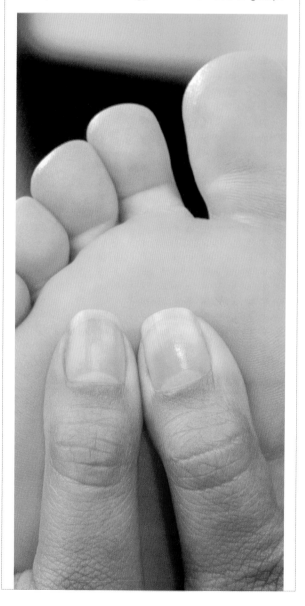

Alexander technique

The Alexander technique is named for Frederick Matthias Alexander, an Australian-English actor who believed in a link between posture, body movement and physical problems. Using the Alexander technique, you learn to become more aware of your posture and body movements.

But unlike other approaches to movement, such as yoga or Pilates, the Alexander technique isn't a set of exercises. Instead, it's a way to heighten your awareness of how you move, to improve your coordination and help you become a more intelligent exerciser. The Alexander technique is used to relieve pain, prevent injury and improve function.

Our take

The Alexander technique is quite popular. For back and neck pain, current evidence shows that it may be helpful, but for other areas, there's not enough research to support its use. Though there are limited data available as to its effectiveness, the risks are minimal. If you think it may help improve your coordination or relieve symptoms such as chronic pain, discuss it with your health care team.

What the research says

In many cases, not enough good-quality research has been conducted to confirm how effective the Alexander technique is for the health conditions it's used to treat. Of the studies that have been done so far, this is what researchers have found.

Pain
A study of about 500 adults showed that the Alexander technique reduced neck pain when compared to typical care. A study of nearly 600 adults with recurrent low back pain found that the Alexander technique helped reduce the number of days that the people studied experienced their back pain.

Mobility and fall risk
A study of 120 visually impaired adults over the age of 50 showed that this approach may improve mobility and help reduce fall risk.

Other conditions
Other areas that have been studied include balance, back pain, chronic pain from the temporomandibular joint (TMJ), Parkinson's disease and lung function. Better-designed studies are necessary to determine the effectiveness of the Alexander technique in treating these and other disorders.

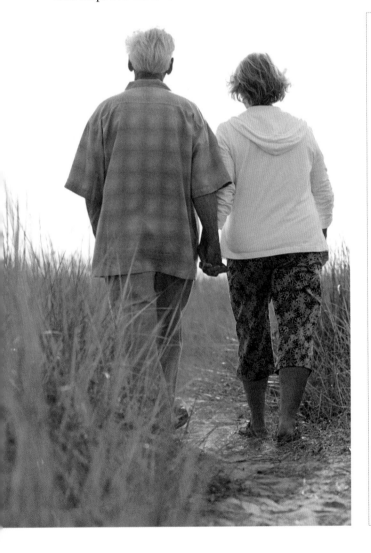

Feldenkrais method

The Feldenkrais method uses gentle movements to develop increased flexibility and coordination. Though similar to yoga, the Feldenkrais method doesn't strive for correct positions, but instead aims for more dexterous, painless and efficient body movements. The goal is to create an awareness and quality of movement through body feedback rather than predefined postures. In group classes, which may be part of a physical or occupational therapy session, the instructor leads you through a sequence of movements — sitting in a chair, lying down or standing — that progress in range and complexity.

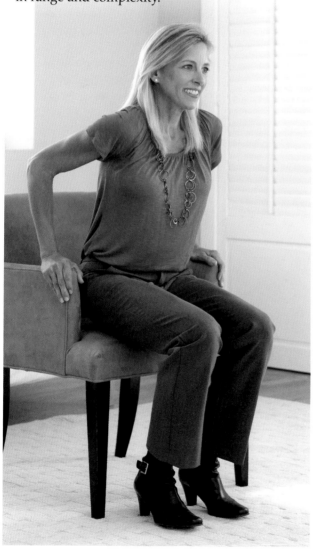

Our take

Similar to the Alexander technique, this form of movement therapy poses little risk. If you think it may help improve a musculo-skeletal problem or symptoms of another condition, go ahead and give it a try. As for its effectiveness, there's not enough research available to reach any definitive conclusions.

What the research says

As with other types of integrative medicine, the Feldenkrais method is not seen as a cure for disease but is likely to be recommended for use alongside conventional medical treatments. The Feldenkrais method has been used to treat a variety of illnesses and disorders, including chronic pain, stress-related conditions, multiple sclerosis, back and neck pain, muscle spasms, and fibromy-algia. But in all cases, more research is needed to verify whether it's effective. Here are some current research findings.

Parkinson's disease
In a small study of adults between ages 50 and 70 with Parkinson's disease, Feldenkrais-based exercises done twice a week seemed to improve quality of life.

Neck, shoulder pain
In another small study, this time of women in their 30s, 40s and 50s who had chronic neck and shoulder pain, those who used the Feldenkrais method said they felt less pain.

Mobility in older adults
A small group of adults in their 70s who took part in a five-week Feldenkrais program seemed to improve their balance and mobility by participating in the program three times a week.

Healing touch

Healing touch is a noninvasive technique that uses the power of touch to influence a person's energy. The goal of healing touch is to improve physical, mental, emotional and spiritual health by helping the person to heal him- or herself. It's similar to therapeutic touch and reiki.

During a healing touch session, the practitioner first moves his or her hands a few inches above the recipient's body. This is done to assess the recipient's energy condition. Then the practitioner gently touches the recipient at various energy points on the body in a way that's designed to move energy through the practitioner to the recipient, strengthening and reorienting the recipient's energy flow within and surrounding the body. The goal is to promote the body's self-healing processes by opening blocked or congested flow of energy. Some people who have undergone healing touch have responded that the treatment resulted in having a more positive mood, lowered pain, reduced anxiety or an improved sense of well-being. A typical session lasts 20 to 30 minutes.

Proponents of healing touch claim that it's effective in treating stress-related problems and heart disease, enhancing the immune system, aiding in recovery from surgery, deepening spiritual connections, supporting cancer care, and decreasing pain. But so far, there's no hard data to confirm this.

Our take

It's understood that people believe that the health benefits from healing relaxation are good for health and wellness.

However, beyond relaxation, there's limited scientific evidence that healing touch improves health, even though it's used for a variety of medical conditions. With this said, there's little risk in healing touch, so whether to try the therapy is up to you, based on how closely it fits with your personal beliefs.

What the research says

Many small studies of healing touch have suggested it's effective in treating a variety of conditions. In a recent study, researchers found that nurses who deliver healing touch find benefit in the practice just as did those who received the therapy. Another study found that children who are hospitalized on an ongoing basis also benefit from receiving healing touch therapy. And although more study is needed, preliminary research shows that healing touch is effective in treating pain, anxiety and fatigue, as well as providing relaxation benefits to those who have undergone outpatient surgery and various types of surgery and medical procedures.

There is some impressive anecdotal evidence that healing touch works. However, more study is needed to confirm these findings.

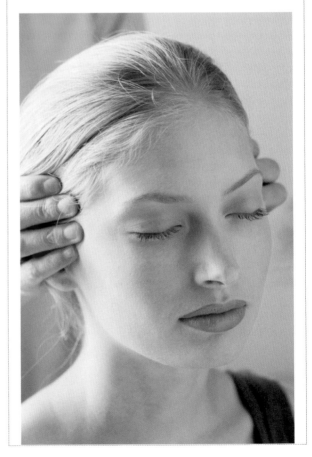

Reiki

Reiki (RAY-kee) is made up of the Japanese words *rei*, which means universal spirit, and *ki* (or *qi*), which means life force energy. As with other energy therapies, practitioners of reiki believe that disturbances in the body's energy systems can cause illness, and that by improving the flow and balance of energy, disease can be treated and health maintained.

The practitioner delivers reiki therapy through his or her hands with the goal of raising the amount of *ki* in and around the recipient. There are many forms of reiki.

A reiki session typically lasts 30 to 90 minutes. During a reiki session, the fully clothed recipient either sits or lies down. The practitioner's hands are placed either on or a few inches above the recipient's body. There are between 12 and 15 different reiki hand positions. Each position is held until the practitioner feels that the flow of energy has slowed or stopped, usually between two to five minutes.

Recipients sometimes describe a deep sense of relaxation after a session, accompanied by a feeling of well-being. They also report sensations of warmth, tingling and sleepiness, and feelings of refreshment.

Reiki is used to treat stress, pain, anxiety, fatigue, nausea from chemotherapy and depression, as well as enhance well-being.

Our take

Similar to healing touch, the benefits associated with reiki may come from its ability to help promote relaxation. There's little, if any, health risk from the therapy. But there's also little evidence that it can effectively treat specific conditions. It's up to you if you think it's worth giving a try.

What the research says

Reiki is touted for the treatment of many diseases and conditions. However, research is limited. Some studies show that reiki may have some effect on blood pressure and heart rates. Initial studies also support the use of reiki as possible therapy in conditions relating to pain, stress, anxiety and mood.

Integrative therapy for common conditions

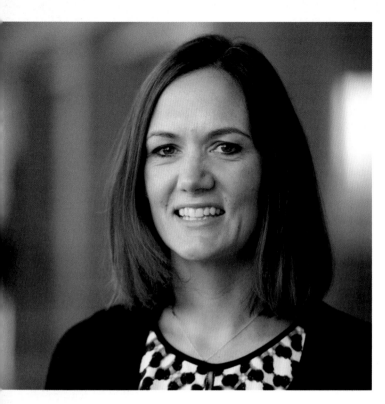

Denise M. Millstine, M.D.
Internal Medicine

Dr. Millstine works in the Women's Health Center at Mayo Clinic in Scottsdale, Arizona, and is a faculty member of the Arizona Center for Integrative Medicine at the University of Arizona in Tucson, Arizona.

A visit with Dr. Millstine

Over time, everyone will experience medical conditions and symptoms. Today's health care system directs people to bring these issues to primary care providers who are trained in medications, procedures and therapy used to reverse, stabilize or improve health conditions.

For example, suppose your hands ache from arthritis and you're unable to sleep. Your primary care provider, trained in conventional medicine, may prescribe two or more medications. A health care provider trained in integrative medicine, however, will consider a broader realm of therapies. Alongside medication, an integrative medicine specialist may also suggest dietary changes, movement practices, mind-body techniques, acupuncture, and supplements or botanicals.

This is one example of how integrative medicine focuses on optimizing health and treating chronic health issues, all by emphasizing several areas of wellness, including diet, physical activity, stress reduction and maintaining connectedness.

Scientific knowledge showing safety and effectiveness of integrative medicine is still unfolding. However, research is growing rapidly. The challenge is to find treatments that are most likely to be beneficial and least likely to be harmful, while avoiding those that are riskier and less likely to help. That's where your health care team can help.

This section reviews eight common conditions for which research is strong in terms of integrative medicine. You'll find both conventional and integrative options discussed for each condition. You'll learn about the current evidence and recommendations, as well as cautionary notes when needed.

By following the same approach with other conditions, you should be able to develop a sound approach to evaluating new therapies with your health care team as they arise.

Wishing you good health!

Arthritis

When you think of arthritis, you likely think of pain and stiffness in joints. And you'd be right on the money. Those are typical symptoms of osteoarthritis and rheumatoid arthritis, the two most common forms of arthritis (there are actually more than 100 forms).

Arthritis is the leading cause of disability in the United States. More than 50 million Americans have been diagnosed with some form of arthritis, and by the year 2040, some experts predict that doctors will diagnose more than 78 million people with some form of arthritis.

Osteoarthritis is commonly known as wear-and-tear arthritis. It involves the wearing away of the tough, lubricated cartilage that normally cushions the ends of bones in your joints. Rheumatoid arthritis results from an abnormal immune system response that causes inflammation of the lining of the joints.

Arthritis affects people of all ages, but it's most common among older adults. Women, possibly because of female hormones, are at higher risk of rheumatoid arthritis than are men.

White people are more likely to get arthritis than are black people, Asians, Hispanics and other minority populations. In addition, people who are more than 10 pounds overweight are at increased risk, especially of arthritis of the knees. Past joint injury also can increase risk of osteoarthritis.

Conventional treatment for osteoarthritis

There's no known cure for osteoarthritis, but treatments can help to reduce pain and maintain joint movement. Conventional treatment typically involves a combination of therapies that may include medication, self-care, physical therapy and occupational therapy. In some cases, surgical procedures may be necessary.

Medications

Medications are used to treat the pain and mild inflammation of osteoarthritis and to improve the function of your joints. They include both topical medications and oral medications. Nonprescription topical pain relievers include Aspercreme, Icy Hot, Bengay, Biofreeze and various formulations containing capsaicin, a cream made from hot chili (cayenne) peppers.

Nonprescription medications such as acetaminophen (Tylenol, others), ibuprofen (Advil, Motrin IB, others) and naproxen sodium (Aleve) may be sufficient to treat milder osteoarthritis, but stronger prescription medications also are available. These include tramadol (Ultram, others), painkillers and various antidepressants.

Occasionally, your doctor may suggest injecting a joint space with a corticosteroid to relieve pain and swelling. Injecting hyaluronic acid derivatives into knee joints (visco-supplementation) also can relieve pain from osteoarthritis. Finally, prolotherapy is one more option for treating symptoms of osteoarthritis. Prolotherapy involves injecting an irritant solution into joints, ligaments and tendons. While it's been in use for many years, researchers and medical experts aren't sure yet how well it improves symptoms.

Surgery or other procedures

Surgical procedures can help relieve disability and pain caused by osteoarthritis. Procedures include joint replacement, arthroscopic lavage and debridement to remove debris from a joint, bone repositioning to help correct deformities, and bone fusion to increase stability and reduce pain.

Self-care

You can relieve much of the discomfort associated with osteoarthritis through healthy-living strategies and self-care techniques. Strategies you can try include:

- Exercising regularly to maintain mobility and range of motion
- Reaching and maintaining a healthy weight to help reduce stress on your joints

- Eating a healthy diet to help control your weight and decrease inflammation
- Applying heat to ease pain and relax tense, painful muscles
- Applying cold to dull the sensation of occasional flare-ups

In addition, choosing comfortable, cushioned footwear is important if you have arthritis in your weight-bearing joints or back. And, it's important to take your medications as recommended to keep pain from increasing.

Complementary and integrative treatment

Several integrative therapies may help relieve the pain of osteoarthritis.

Glucosamine and chondroitin

Glucosamine is a dietary supplement derived from oyster and crab shells. It's a synthetic version of an amino sugar the body produces to preserve joint health. Chondroitin is a dietary supplement derived from cow and shark cartilage and other sources. The two are often used in combination.

Some research shows that glucosamine and chondroitin can help decrease pain and improve joint function in osteoarthritis. In terms of rheumatoid arthritis, limited evidence shows that it may help reduce pain. Learn more about what researchers have to say about glucosamine and chondroitin for treating arthritis on page 107.

Acupuncture

During acupuncture, hair-thin needles are inserted into your skin at specific spots on your body. This therapy has been shown to reduce many types of pain, including pain caused by some types of arthritis. Some studies show that acupuncture can relieve pain and improve function in people who have knee osteoarthritis. Learn more about acupuncture, including how to find an experienced practitioner, starting on page 94.

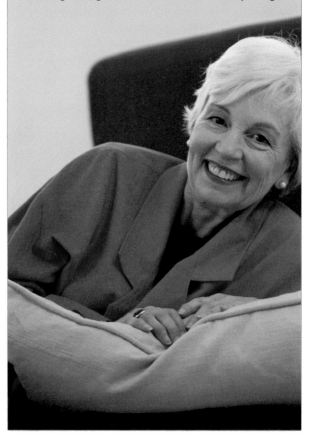

Coping skills are important

Because osteoarthritis can affect your everyday activities and overall quality of life, coping strategies are an important element of dealing with the disease, no matter which conventional or integrative therapies you use.

Coping strategies include keeping a positive attitude so that you're in charge of your disease, rather than vice versa, knowing when to limit activities, using assistive devices and avoiding grasping actions that can strain finger joints.

Strategies also include spreading the weight of an object over several joints when lifting, such as using both hands to lift a heavy pan, maintaining good posture to evenly distribute your weight, and using your strongest muscles and large joints (for example, leaning into a heavy door to open it rather than pushing it with your hands).

An occupational therapist also can help you in selecting the right assistive devices for daily living.

Tai chi and yoga

The slow, stretching movements associated with yoga and tai chi may help improve joint flexibility and range of motion in people with some types of arthritis. Avoid movements that cause pain. Learn more about tai chi and yoga on page 29.

SAMe

Commercially available SAMe is a synthetic version of a compound that occurs naturally in human tissue. Some research shows that this dietary supplement can reduce the pain of osteoarthritis as well as nonsteroidal anti-inflammatory drugs (NSAIDs) do. SAMe is thought to stimulate cartilage growth and repair, as well as increase cartilage thickness.

You may need to take SAMe for several weeks before you experience relief from symptoms. Side effects can include gas, vomiting, diarrhea, headache and nausea. It's also important to note that SAMe can negatively interact with antidepressant medications and shouldn't be taken if you have bipolar disorder and are taking monoamine oxidase inhibitors (MAOIs). It may also worsen Parkinson's disease.

Ginger extract

Although some research suggests that ginger may modestly improve pain in osteoarthritis, there's not enough evidence to say if it can help improve symptoms of rheumatoid arthritis. More study is needed. Learn more about ginger on page 122.

Cat's claw

Studies suggest that taking a specific freeze-dried botanical cat's claw extract orally may help relieve osteoarthritis-related knee pain. Other research suggests that a specific combination supplement containing cat's claw may help reduce pain and stiffness and improve function in osteoarthritis. Some research also shows that when taken orally, one cat's claw extract may modestly improve pain and swelling related to rheumatoid arthritis.

When cat's claw is taken in small amounts, few side effects have been reported. Ask your doctor which type and how much to take.

Devil's claw

A traditional herb used in South Africa, devil's claw has been said to relieve pain and inflammation. A review of research on the use of devil's claw for arthritis shows mixed results. Some studies show that it may help reduce pain associated with osteoarthritis, while other research showed no improvement in symptoms.

Avocado and soybean oil

Researchers have found that components of avocado and soybean oils may improve pain and function slightly, but more research is needed. This nutritional supplement is a mixture of avocado and soybean oils.

Fish oil

Several randomized controlled trials show that fish oil supplements can reduce morning stiffness and joint tenderness when taken regularly for up to three months. Researchers are not sure yet of the effects of fish oil when taken for longer than three months.

Fish oil may even reduce the need for nonsteroidal anti-inflammatory drugs. However, research quality isn't strong, so more study is needed. Learn more about fish oil on page 106.

Turmeric

Clinical research shows that the curcumin in turmeric may reduce morning stiffness and joint swelling. Learn more about turmeric on page 117.

Magnets

Although they remain popular, there's little evidence to support the use of magnets for

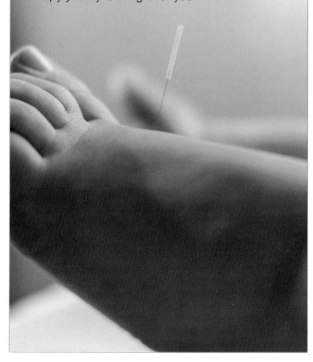

arthritis. Side effects appear to be rare, but magnets can disrupt implantable defibrillators and pacemakers. Magnets should be avoided in these cases, as well as during pregnancy.

Conventional treatment for rheumatoid arthritis

Treatment for rheumatoid arthritis typically involves a combination of self-care techniques similar to those used for osteoarthritis (see page 150) and medications. Sometimes, surgery or other procedures may be necessary.

Medications

Medications for rheumatoid arthritis can relieve its symptoms and slow or halt its progression.

Nonsteroidal anti-inflammatory drugs (NSAIDs), such as ibuprofen (Advil, Motrin IB) and naproxen sodium (Aleve), are available as an over-the-counter option. Corticosteroids such as prednisone reduce inflammation and pain and slow joint damage.

Disease-modifying antirheumatic drugs (DMARDs), such as methotrexate (Trexall, Otrex-up, Rasuvo), leflunomide (Arava), hydroxychloroquine (Plaquenil) and sulfasalazine (Azulfidine), can slow the progression of rheumatoid arthritis and save joints and other tissues from permanent damage.

Also used are biologic agents, also known as biologic response modifiers. This newer class of DMARDs includes abatacept (Orencia), adalimumab (Humira), anakinra (Kineret), certolizumab (Cimzia), etanercept (Enbrel), golimumab (Simponi), infliximab (Remicade), rituximab (Rituxan), tocilizumab (Actemra) and tofacitinib (Xeljanz). These drugs can target parts of the immune system that trigger the inflammation that causes joint and tissue damage.

Surgery and other procedures

If joint destruction is too severe, joint replacement can often help restore joint function, reduce pain or correct a deformity.

Complementary and integrative treatment

Fish oil

Some preliminary studies have found that fish oil supplements may reduce rheumatoid arthritis pain and stiffness. Side effects can include nausea, belching and a fishy taste in the mouth. Fish oil can interfere with medications, so check with your doctor first. Learn more about fish oil supplements on page 106.

Plant oils

Preliminary evidence shows that the seeds of evening primrose, borage and black currant contain a type of fatty acid that may help with rheumatoid arthritis pain and morning stiffness. Side effects may include nausea, diarrhea and gas. Some plant oils can cause liver damage or interfere with medications, so check with your doctor first to ensure that they're safe for you.

Turmeric

Although reliable human research is lacking, turmeric is often used to treat rheumatoid arthritis and osteoarthritis because of its anti-inflammatory properties. Learn more about turmeric on page 117.

Tai chi

This movement therapy involves gentle exercises and stretches combined with deep breathing. Small studies have found that tai chi may reduce rheumatoid arthritis pain. When led by a knowledgeable instructor, tai chi is safe, but avoid movements that cause pain. Learn more about tai chi on page 29.

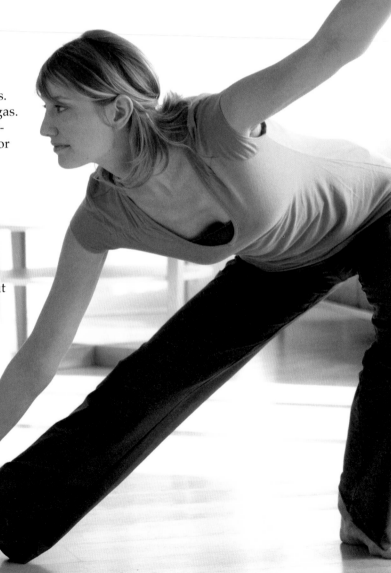

Our take

The strongest evidence in integrative medicine for rheumatoid arthritis is in using fish oil. Although taking fish oil supplements can carry some risks (see page 106 for more information), several randomized controlled trials have shown that taking fish oil can help improve symptoms of rheumatoid arthritis, including morning stiffness and joint tenderness, when it's taken regularly for up to three months.

Chronic fatigue syndrome

Chronic fatigue syndrome is a complicated disorder characterized by extreme fatigue that doesn't improve with bed rest and may worsen with physical or mental activity.

Of all the chronic illnesses in this section, chronic fatigue syndrome is one of the most mysterious. Unlike infections, chronic fatigue syndrome has no clear cause. Unlike conditions such as diabetes or anemia, there's essentially nothing to measure. And unlike conditions such as heart disease, there are relatively few treatment options. But medical experts do feel that they have an explanation for syndromes like this: a concept called *central sensitization*. (Learn more starting on page 180.)

Chronic fatigue syndrome may occur after an infection such as a cold or viral syndrome. It can start during or shortly after a period of high stress or come on gradually without any clear starting point or any obvious cause.

A flu-like condition, chronic fatigue syndrome can drain your energy and sometimes last for years. People previously healthy and full of energy may experience a variety of symptoms, including extreme fatigue and headaches, as well as difficulty concentrating and painful joints, muscles and lymph nodes.

Women are diagnosed with chronic fatigue syndrome two to four times as often as are men. However, it's unclear whether chronic fatigue syndrome affects women more often or if women report it to their doctors more often than do men.

Signs and symptoms

In addition to persistent fatigue not caused by other known medical conditions, medical experts have confirmed that chronic fatigue syndrome has several other possible primary signs and symptoms. These are:

- Fatigue
- Loss of memory or concentration
- Sore throat that is frequent or recurs
- Enlarged lymph nodes in your neck or armpits
- Unexplained muscle soreness
- Headache of a new type, pattern or severity

- Pain that moves from one joint to another without swelling or redness
- Sleep that doesn't feel refreshing
- Extreme exhaustion lasting more than 24 hours after physical or mental exercise

According to the Centers for Disease Control and Prevention (CDC), a person meets the diagnostic criteria of chronic fatigue syndrome when unexplained persistent fatigue occurs for six months in a row or more and at least four of these signs and symptoms are present.

Conventional treatment

There's no specific conventional treatment for chronic fatigue syndrome because it affects people in different ways. Doctors aim to relieve symptoms by using a combination of treatments specific to a set of symptoms.

Treatments for symptoms of chronic fatigue syndrome may include:

Lifestyle changes

Your doctor may encourage you to pace your activity level. This may save your energy for essential activities at home or work and help you cut back on less important activities.

Your doctor may also help you make changes in your sleeping routine to help you improve your sleep quality.

Gradual but steady exercise

Often, with the help of a physical therapist, your health care team may recommend that you begin an exercise program in which you gradually increase your physical activity.

Taking this approach to exercise can help prevent or decrease the muscle weakness caused by prolonged inactivity. In addition, exercise improves your energy level and sleep.

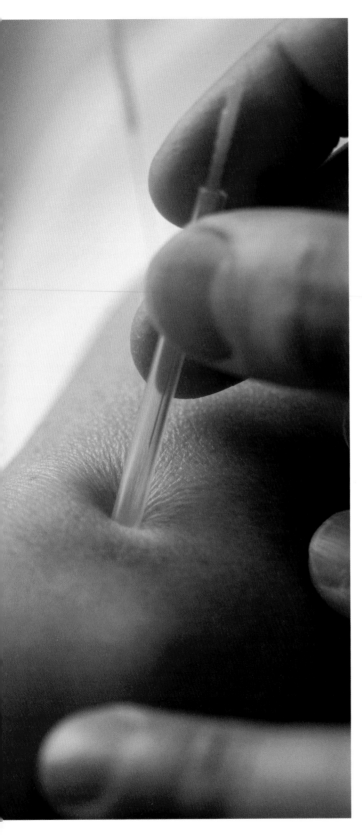

Counseling

Talking with a counselor can help you figure out options to work around some of the limitations that chronic fatigue syndrome imposes on you. Self-management strategies and cognitive behavioral therapy — in which you work to identify and cope with specific challenges — are among the most helpful. Ultimately, the goal of counseling is to help you feel more in control of your life, which can improve your outlook dramatically.

Antidepressants

Many people who have chronic fatigue syndrome are also depressed. Treating your depression can make it easier for you to cope with the problems associated with chronic fatigue syndrome. Low doses of some antidepressants also can help improve sleep and relieve pain.

Treatment of existing pain

Acetaminophen (Tylenol, others) or nonsteroidal anti-inflammatory drugs (NSAIDs) such as ibuprofen (Advil, Motrin IB, others) and naproxen sodium (Aleve) may be helpful to reduce pain and fever.

Treatment of allergy-like symptoms

Antihistamines such as fexofenadine (Allegra) and cetirizine (Zyrtec) and decongestants that contain pseudoephedrine (Sudafed) may relieve allergy-like symptoms such as runny nose.

Treatment of low blood pressure (hypotension)

The drugs fludrocortisone and midodrine may be useful for certain people with chronic fatigue syndrome whose blood pressure drops far below normal levels.

Some medications can cause side effects or adverse reactions that may be worse than the symptoms of chronic fatigue syndrome. Talk to your doctor before starting any treatment for chronic fatigue syndrome.

Complementary and integrative treatment

Because the causes of chronic fatigue syndrome are not clear, an integrative approach to treatment involves addressing a variety of possible factors.

It's difficult to know if integrative therapies can help ease symptoms of chronic fatigue syndrome, in part because the symptoms of chronic fatigue syndrome often are linked to mood and can vary. However, certain integrative strategies can help ease the pain associated with chronic fatigue syndrome.

Acupuncture

Researchers list acupuncture among many different types of integrative medicine that can be used to help treat chronic fatigue syndrome. Research on acupuncture for chronic fatigue syndrome is limited and ongoing, but some studies suggest that it may help improve a person's ability to manage this condition.

In one study of 150 participants in four different hospitals, researchers found that 10 sessions of acupuncture given over four weeks — in addition to standard medical care — helped improve symptoms of fatigue. Learn more about acupuncture on page 94.

Spinal manipulation

Although evidence is lacking on how well spinal manipulation can help treat symptoms of chronic fatigue syndrome, it is a therapy that's sometimes used to treat this condition. Learn more about spinal manipulation on page 76.

Massage

Massage is yet another type of integrative therapy that's used to help treat chronic fatigue syndrome. Some researchers believe that massage is helpful in part because it helps improve how well a person feels he or she can manage the condition.

Studies show that massage can offer positive effects for people managing chronic fatigue syndrome, but more research and better quality studies are needed. Learn more about massage on page 82.

Yoga

As with many other types of integrative therapy used to help treat chronic fatigue syndrome, more study is needed on how well practicing yoga can help people manage symptoms of this condition.

As with massage and other types of complementary therapies, yoga is thought to help improve a person's ability to manage the symptoms of this condition. Learn more about yoga on page 29.

Tai chi

Tai chi is another example of integrative medicine that's often useful for managing chronic fatigue syndrome — and, in particular, a person's confidence in being able to manage symptoms of this condition.

More research on tai chi and its effects on chronic fatigue syndrome are needed. Learn more about tai chi on page 29.

Meditation

A common type of complementary technique for managing symptoms of chronic fatigue syndrome, meditation has undergone some study in terms of its usefulness in helping treat this condition.

Two randomized controlled trials suggest that mindfulness-based stress reduction, paired with qi gong, was helpful in treating anxiety associated with chronic fatigue syndrome.

Other research concludes that although more study is needed on the benefits of meditation for chronic fatigue syndrome, meditation shows some benefit as a generally safe and relatively low-cost treatment to try. Learn more about meditation, with instructions, starting on page 56.

Fatigue is a common and vexing problem for many people. At Mayo Clinic, physicians always ask patients to look for common causes of fatigue first. Exercise, sleep and diet can be common culprits to consider correcting before trying other approaches. But if fatigue is still a major issue despite lifestyle changes, as well as conventional treatment and care, an integrative approach is a reasonable next step.

"I usually start by making sure my patients are practicing a mind-body therapy at least 30 minutes — and preferably 60 minutes — a day. I also often suggest a trial of acupuncture, as well as massage for those who also have muscle pain," says Brent A. Bauer, M.D., medical editor, *Mayo Clinic Guide to Integrative Medicine,* and director of research in Integrative Medicine and Health at Mayo Clinic in Rochester, Minnesota. "But every one of us is unique, so finding what works best for you may take some patience, as well as a little trial and error. Eventually, I'd say that 80 percent of my patients see a substantial improvement in their fatigue once they find the combination of conventional and integrative approaches that fits them best."

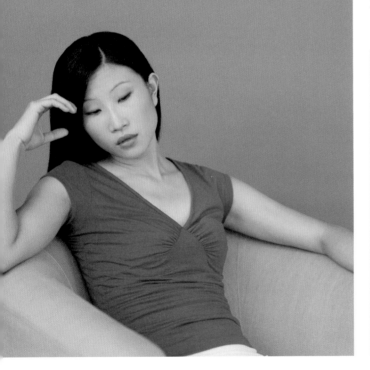

Muscle relaxation and other relaxation techniques

Only a few studies have focused on using relaxation techniques to help treat chronic fatigue syndrome. Of those, one randomized controlled trial shows that these exercises, when done over 12 weeks, may help reduce fatigue and improve functioning.

Other studies suggest using relaxation techniques with other types of treatment because not enough research shows that relaxation techniques are effective on their own. Learn more about relaxation exercises on page 43.

Healing touch

Healing touch is an energy therapy that helps balance your physical, mental, emotional and spiritual well-being when performed by a trained professional. It works with your energy field to support your body's natural ability to heal itself.

Therapeutic touch is sometimes used to help relieve symptoms of chronic fatigue syndrome, although not much study has been done to prove its benefits. Learn more about healing touch on page 146.

A note about depression and anxiety

Chronic fatigue is not a form of depression, nor is it an anxiety disorder. However, depression and anxiety often go hand in hand with chronic fatigue, just as they do with many other long-term medical conditions. It is natural to feel discouraged or anxious about fatigue. But, if symptoms of depression or anxiety linger, or become severe, talk to your doctor.

Depression and anxiety can be treated effectively, and studies have shown that treating them may reduce fatigue or make fatigue easier to manage.

Chronic pain

Everyone experiences pain, and you likely know that there are two different types of pain: acute and chronic.

Acute pain is severe or sudden but resolves after a certain amount of time. An illness, injury or surgery can be a cause of acute pain. Pain medication provides relief while your body heals.

Chronic pain is different from acute pain and is considered a health condition in itself. Sometimes, chronic pain follows an illness or an injury that appears to have healed. It can also be related to long-standing conditions such as arthritis. Other times, chronic pain develops for no reason that you or your health care team can find.

Whatever the cause, the emotional fallout of chronic pain can make you hurt even more. Anxiety or depression can magnify unpleasant sensations, and disrupted sleep may leave you feeling fatigued and helpless.

Conventional treatment

Chronic pain can be challenging to manage, but a variety of conventional treatment options can help. They include:

Medication

Sometimes, over-the-counter pain relievers or medicated creams or gels are effective. For more severe pain, your doctor may give you a prescription pain medication, such as tramadol (Ultram, Conzip). Some people find relief with tricyclic antidepressants such as nortriptyline (Pamelor) or amitriptyline. Anti-seizure drugs such as gabapentin (Gralise, Neurontin) or pregabalin (Lyrica) may relieve some types of chronic pain as well.

Injection therapy

Instead of prescribing pills to control chronic pain, your doctor might inject medication directly into the affected area. Such injections are usually a combination of a numbing agent (local anesthet-

ic), which provides immediate relief, and a corticosteroid, which reduces inflammation.

Nerve stimulation

Various devices use electric impulses to help block or mask the feeling of pain. With transcutaneous electrical nerve stimulation (TENS), a portable, battery-powered unit delivers an electric impulse through electrodes placed on the affected area. Spinal cord and peripheral nerve stimulators are implanted beneath the skin with electrodes placed near the spinal cord. A hand-held unit allows you to control the level of stimulation.

Medication pumps

Implantable medication pumps supply pain medication directly into the spinal fluid. To replenish the pump, drugs are injected through the skin into a small port at the center of the pump. This less common approach must be managed by a pain specialist.

Physical and occupational therapy

Stretching and strengthening exercises can improve your strength and flexibility. Sometimes learning new ways to handle daily activities can minimize the pain.

Counseling

Cognitive behavioral therapy can help you manage your emotional response to chronic pain, as well as identify patterns of thought or behavior that may aggravate your pain.

Exercise

Exercise can prompt your body to release endorphins, chemicals that block pain signals from reaching your brain. Exercise can also help you build strength, increase flexibility, improve sleep quality and boost your energy level. In addition, it can improve mood and protect your heart and blood vessels. If you have chronic pain, talk to your doctor before starting an exercise program.

Complementary and integrative treatment

Various complementary therapies can offer relief from chronic pain.

Acupuncture

This traditional Chinese therapy involves the insertion of fine needles into the skin at certain points to restore proper energy flow in the body. There's strong evidence that acupuncture can relieve many different kinds of pain, including low back and neck pain, osteoarthritis, headache, fibromyalgia, and pain after surgery. Acupuncture is generally safe. Learn more about acupuncture starting on page 94.

Guided imagery

Visualization, game playing and storytelling are all examples of guided imagery techniques. The goal is to help people visualize positive outcomes for issues they're dealing with. Guided imagery may alter breathing, heart rate and blood pressure. With pain, it's been shown to reduce postoperative pain and cancer pain, but more research is needed to confirm how effective it truly is in helping manage pain. Learn more about guided imagery on page 64.

Guided imagery is generally considered safe. However, it could interact with certain mental conditions, so use it only with professional guidance if you have mental health issues.

Massage

A growing body of literature is beginning to validate the many benefits of massage therapy.

Studies suggest it can help decrease headache pain, fibromyalgia pain, back pain, neck and shoulder pain, myofascial pain syndrome, and temporomandibular joint (TMJ) pain. Learn more about massage therapy starting on page 82.

Biofeedback

Biofeedback is often used as part of a comprehensive treatment plan for chronic pain. Studies show it may improve symptoms of headache, anxiety, stress, fibromyalgia, irritable bowel syndrome, and TMJ pain. Learn more about biofeedback on page 66.

Hypnotherapy

There's evidence that hypnotherapy may help relieve pain associated with cancer, irritable bowel syndrome, fibromyalgia, TMJ problems, dental procedures and headaches. Learn more about hypnotherapy on page 69.

Music therapy

Music therapy has been shown to raise pain thresholds, improve mood and provide relaxation, and has been effective in reducing pain from cancer, burns, osteoarthritis and surgery, among other conditions.

Music therapists are trained to adapt music therapy to specific needs and situations. Learn more about music therapy on page 50.

Meditation

Originally meant to help deepen understanding of the sacred and mystical forces of life, meditation is commonly used these days for relaxation and stress reduction. Some research shows that it may be a helpful way to manage pain. However, meditation is often used with other treatments and therapies, so scientifically, its benefit as a standalone therapy in treating and relieving chronic pain isn't clear. Learn more about meditation on starting on page 56.

Tai chi

Often described as meditation in motion, tai chi promotes serenity through gentle, flowing movements. Some research suggests that it may help reduce joint pain by strengthening muscles and improving joint flexibility.

Although it has been suggested that tai chi can be an effective way to manage chronic pain, not enough research has been done to show that it's effective. And for some people, tai chi may cause harm. Learn more about tai chi on page 29.

Supplements

Several dietary supplements are often used to help manage chronic pain. Fish oil, for example, can help improve morning stiffness and relieve joint stiffness in rheumatoid arthritis. Glucosamine and chondroitin are used to treat osteoarthritis. Learn more about these supplements starting on page 107.

Conflicting or unclear evidence

In healing (therapeutic) touch, practitioners hold their hands close to a person to sense and manipulate the person's energy field. It's said that healing touch helps your body heal itself. Evidence is limited regarding effect of healing touch, but many people report that they feel very relaxed after a healing touch session. Pending more studies, at this point it is seen as safe to try, but it may not help.

Similarly, magnet therapy is popular but has very little in the way of scientific evidence to support its use as a pain treatment. In addition, the use of magnets can pose risks in a number of different situations. They can disrupt implantable defibrillators and pacemakers and should be avoided during pregnancy.

And finally, the Feldenkrais method, which uses gentle movements to develop increased flexibility and coordination, has been thought to help reduce neck and shoulder pain, but there hasn't been enough research done to say for sure. Learn more about the Feldenkrais method on page 145.

Our take

Of the integrative therapies often used to help treat, manage and relieve pain, acupuncture shows the most promise. A clear majority of the studies that have been conducted on acupuncture and pain after surgery, for example, show that it offers pain-relieving benefits.

There's also good evidence to support the use of spinal manipulation when used appropriately, as well as music therapy and physical therapy.

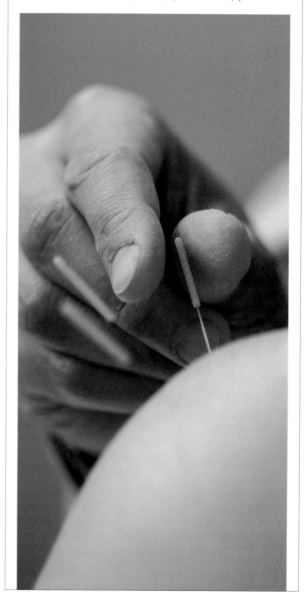

Fibromyalgia

You hurt all over and frequently feel exhausted. Even after numerous tests, your doctor can't seem to find anything specifically wrong with you. If this sounds familiar, you may have fibromyalgia.

Fibromyalgia is a chronic condition characterized by fatigue, widespread pain, cognitive difficulties often referred to as "fibro fog" that make it difficult to focus, and other signs and symptoms, including depression, headaches, and pain or cramping in the lower abdomen. Fibromyalgia affects women more often than it does men.

The cause of fibromyalgia is a bit of a mystery. However, as with chronic fatigue syndrome, current thinking centers around a concept called *central sensitization* (see page 182). This theory states that people with fibromyalgia have a lower threshold for pain because of increased sensitivity in the brain to pain signals. Researchers speculate that this oversensitization may be triggered by a range of triggers, including infections, physical trauma or emotional stress. Because fibromyalgia tends to run in families, there may be certain genetic mutations that may make you more susceptible to developing the disorder as well.

Although the intensity of symptoms may vary, they typically never disappear completely. However, fibromyalgia isn't progressive, crippling or life-threatening.

Conventional treatment

In general, treatment for fibromyalgia involves a combination of medication and self-care. The emphasis is on minimizing symptoms and improving general health.

Medications

Medications that can help reduce the pain of fibromyalgia and improve sleep include:

Pain relievers. Over-the-counter pain relievers such as acetaminophen (Tylenol, others), ibuprofen (Advil, Motrin IB, others) or naproxen sodium (Aleve) may be helpful. Your doctor might suggest a prescription pain reliever such as tramadol (Ultram, Conzip).

Antidepressants. Your doctor may prescribe antidepressant medications, such as duloxetine (Cymbalta) and milnacipran (Savella) to help ease pain and fatigue. Your doctor may also prescribe amitriptyline for night-time use to help you sleep.

Anti-seizure drugs

Medications designed to treat epilepsy are often useful in reducing certain types of pain. Gabapentin (Gralise, Neurontin) is sometimes helpful in reducing symptoms, while pregabalin (Lyrica) was the first drug approved by the Food and Drug Administration to treat fibromyalgia.

Self-care

Self-care is critical in the management of fibromyalgia. Here are several steps to take:

Reduce stress. Develop a plan to avoid or limit overexertion and emotional stress. Allow yourself time each day to relax. That may mean learning how to say no without guilt. But try not to change your routine completely. People who quit work or drop all activity tend to do worse than do those who remain active. Try stress management techniques, such as deep-breathing exercises or meditation.

Get enough sleep. Because fatigue is one of the main characteristics of fibromyalgia, getting sufficient sleep is essential. In addition to allotting enough time for sleep, practice good sleep habits, such as going to bed and getting up at the same time each day and limiting daytime napping.

Exercise regularly. At first, exercise may increase your pain. But doing it gradually and regularly often decreases symptoms. Appropriate exercises may include walking, swimming, biking and water aerobics.

If you need additional guidance, a physical therapist can help you develop a home exercise program. Stretching, good posture and relaxation exercises also are helpful.

Follow a healthy diet. Eat healthy foods and limit your caffeine intake. Try to limit your intake of processed foods, sugars and sweeteners.

Pace yourself. Keep your activity on an even level. If you do too much on your good days, you may have more bad days. Moderation means not overdoing it on your good days, but likewise it means not self-limiting or doing too little on the days when symptoms flare.

Make time for enjoyment. Do something that you find enjoyable and fulfilling every day.

Treatment programs

Interdisciplinary treatment programs (see page 193) may help improve fibromyalgia symptoms, including relieving pain. These programs can combine a variety of treatments, such as relaxation techniques, biofeedback, and gentle, graded exercise. Receiving information and learning about chronic pain can be very helpful. There isn't one combination that works best for everybody. Your doctor can create or refer you to a program based on what works best for you.

Complementary and integrative treatment

Several integrative treatments do appear to safely relieve stress and reduce pain, but many practices remain unproved because they haven't been adequately studied. Here's what the latest research shows.

Acupuncture

Results of research done on acupuncture for fibromyalgia are mixed. Some studies indicate that acupuncture helps relieve fibromyalgia symptoms, while others show no benefit. Of the

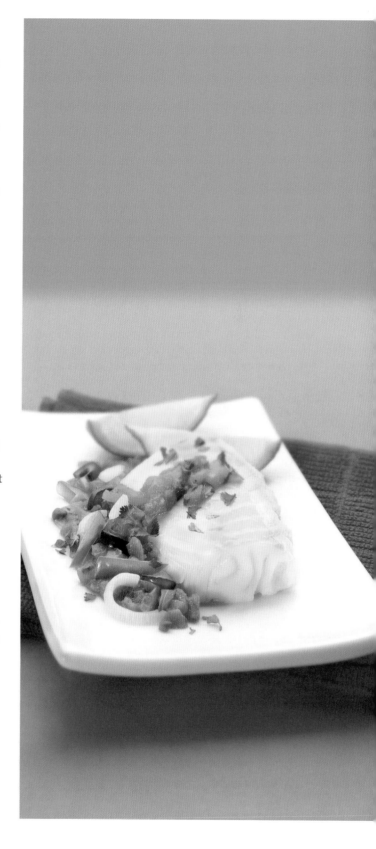

limited evidence that shows it may help, researchers say that people with fibromyalgia who receive acupuncture have less pain and stiffness, and that acupuncture can help improve overall well-being and reduce fatigue. Acupuncture has also been shown to potentially enhance the effects of exercise and medication on pain. However, to date, when it's compared with a simulated version, true acupuncture hasn't been shown to be any more effective in treating fibromyalgia symptoms.

Acupuncture is generally considered to be safe when performed by an experienced practitioner using sterile needles. Learn more about acupuncture starting on page 94.

Massage

Several studies have focused on how well various types of massage therapy can help treat signs and symptoms of fibromyalgia. A small number of studies show that massage may reduce pain, improve symptoms of depression and improve quality of life for people who have fibromyalgia. Most of the studies that have been done show that massage can relieve some symptoms for a short time. However, more research is needed to confirm how much of an effect massage therapy has on this condition. Learn more about massage therapy, including its risks and benefits, starting on page 82.

Moving meditation

Yoga, tai chi and qi gong are all examples of practices that combine meditation, slow movements, deep breathing and relaxation. All of them have been studied to assess their effectiveness in managing fibromyalgia symptoms, but more research is needed to confirm their benefits.

A 2010 study showed that when it was compared with a 12-week wellness education and stretching program, participants in a 12-week tai chi program experienced less pain, better sleep quality, less depression and better quality of life overall. These benefits lasted up to 24 weeks.

Although evidence for qi gong and fibromyalgia is mixed, a 2009 review found that qi gong

may improve fibromyalgia symptoms. And finally, yoga can help you manage stress, which is yet another way to help manage the painful symptoms of fibromyalgia. Learn more about yoga, tai chi, and qi gong on page 29.

Our take

Of all the integrative therapies currently under study for treatment of fibromyalgia, the strongest evidence points to acupuncture as a successful treatment. Several studies suggest that acupuncture may help relieve pain in fibromyalgia. More high-quality studies are needed to confirm these study results.

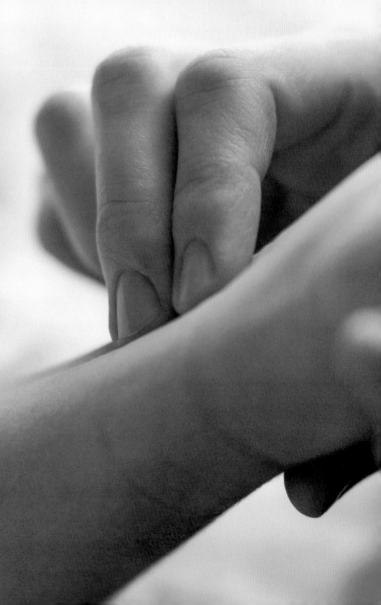

Headache

Although headache pain can be severe, in most cases it's not the result of an underlying disease. The vast majority of headaches are so-called primary headaches. These include migraine and tension headache.

A tension headache is the most common headache, and yet it's not well-understood. A tension headache generally produces a diffuse, mild to moderate pain over the entire head. Many people liken the feeling to having a tight band around their heads. In many cases, there's no clear cause for a tension headache.

Migraines affect more than 36 million Americans — three times as many women as men. A migraine is often disabling. In some cases, these painful headaches are preceded or accompanied by a sensory warning sign (aura), such as flashes of light, blind spots, or tingling on one side of your face or in your arm or leg. A migraine can also be accompanied by other signs and symptoms, such as nausea, vomiting, and extreme sensitivity to light and sound.

Managing headaches is often a balance between fostering healthy habits, finding effective nondrug treatments and using medications appropriately. In addition, a number of preventive, self-care and integrative treatments may help you deal with headache pain.

Conventional treatment

Treatment for headaches depends on the type of headache you have. Here's an overview of treatment options for two main types of headaches: tension headaches and migraines.

Tension headaches: Pain-relieving medications

A variety of medications, both nonprescription and prescription, are available for treating tension headaches. You may find fast, effective relief by taking pain relievers such as aspirin, ibuprofen (Advil, Motrin IB, others) or naproxen sodium (Aleve). These medications are inexpensive and

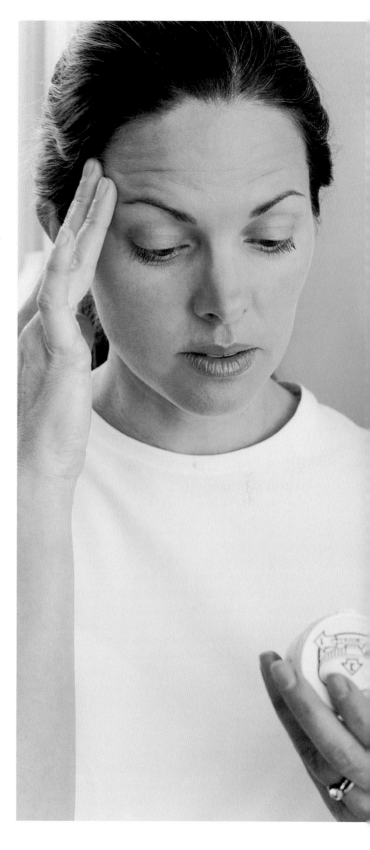

readily available and don't require a prescription from your doctor. People with severe or chronic tension headache may require stronger painkillers or preventive medications. Which drug works best varies from one person to another.

Whether you have episodic or chronic headaches, don't overuse nonprescription medications. Limit your use of painkillers to two days a week. Try to take the medications only when necessary, and use the smallest dose needed to relieve your pain. Overusing pain medications can cause rebound headaches or the development of chronic daily headache, triggering the very symptoms you're trying to stop. In addition, all medications used to treat headache have side effects, some of which may be serious. For prescription medications, follow your doctor's recommendations.

Medications don't cure headaches, and over time, painkillers and other medications may lose their effectiveness. If you take medications regularly, discuss the risks and benefits with your doctor. Also, remember that pain medications aren't a substitute for recognizing and dealing with the stressors that may be causing your headaches.

Migraines: Pain-relieving medications

Pain-relieving medications are taken to stop pain once it has started. For best results, take pain-relieving drugs as soon as you experience signs or symptoms of a migraine. It may help if you rest or sleep in a dark room after taking them. Here are several examples of pain-relieving medications used to treat migraines.

Aspirin, ibuprofen, acetaminophen. Aspirin, ibuprofen (Advil, Motrin IB, others) or acetaminophen (Tylenol, others) may help relieve mild migraines. Drugs marketed specifically for migraines, such as the combination of acetaminophen, aspirin and caffeine (Excedrin Migraine), also may ease moderate migraine pain. They usually aren't effective alone for severe migraines. Note that if they're taken too often or for long periods of time, these medications can lead to ulcers, gastrointestinal bleeding and medication-overuse headaches.

Triptans. These medications are often used in treating migraines. Triptans make blood vessels constrict and block pain pathways in the brain. Triptans effectively relieve the pain and other symptoms that are associated with migraines. They are available in pill, nasal spray and injection form. Triptan medications include sumatriptan (Imitrex), rizatriptan (Maxalt), almotriptan (Axert), naratriptan (Amerge), zolmitriptan (Zomig), frovatriptan (Frova) and eletriptan (Relpax).

Side effects of triptans include reactions at the injection site, nausea, dizziness, drowsiness and muscle weakness. They aren't recommended for people at risk of strokes and heart attacks. A single-tablet combination of sumatriptan and naproxen sodium (Treximet) has proved to be more effective in relieving migraine symptoms than either medication on its own.

Ergots. Ergotamine and caffeine combination drugs (Migergot, Cafergot) are less effective than triptans. Ergots seem most effective in those whose pain lasts for more than 48 hours. Ergots are most effective when taken soon after migraine symptoms start. Ergotamine may worsen nausea and vomiting related to your migraines, and it may also lead to medication-overuse headaches. Dihydroergotamine (D.H.E. 45, Migranal) is an ergot derivative that is more effective and has fewer side effects than ergotamine. It's also less likely to lead to medication-overuse headaches. It's available as a nasal spray and in injection form.

Anti-nausea medications. Medication for nausea is usually combined with other medications. Frequently prescribed medications are chlorpromazine, metoclopramide (Reglan) or prochlorperazine (Compro).

Opioid medications. With the understanding that they are habit-forming, opioid medications, particularly codeine and sometimes hydrocodone, are sometimes used to treat migraine pain when other treatments can't be used or aren't effective.

Glucocorticoids (prednisone, dexamethasone). A glucocorticoid may be used with other medications to improve pain relief. To prevent side effects, glucocorticoids shouldn't be used frequently.

Migraines: Preventive medications

These drugs help reduce or prevent migraines. Choosing a preventive strategy depends on the frequency and severity of your headaches, the degree of disability your headaches cause, and other medical conditions you may have.

You may be a candidate for preventive therapy if you have two or more debilitating attacks a month, if you use pain-relieving medications more than twice a week, if pain-relieving medications aren't helping or if you have uncommon migraines. The most common medications are:

Cardiovascular drugs. Beta blockers, which are commonly used to treat high blood pressure and coronary artery disease, may reduce the frequency and severity of migraines. The beta blockers propranolol (Inderal LA, Innopran XL, others), metoprolol tartrate (Lopressor) and timolol (Betimol) have proved effective for preventing migraines. Other beta blockers are also sometimes used for treatment of migraine. You may not notice improvement in symptoms for several weeks after taking these medications.

If you are older than age 60, use tobacco, or have certain heart or blood vessel conditions, doctors may recommend you take a different medication. Another class of cardiovascular medications (calcium channel blockers) used to treat high blood pressure also may be helpful in preventing migraines and relieving symptoms. Verapamil (Calan, Verelan) is a calcium channel blocker that may help prevent migraines with aura. In addition, the angiotensin-converting enzyme inhibitor lisinopril (Zestril) may be useful in reducing the length and severity of migraines.

Antidepressants. Tricyclic antidepressants may be effective in preventing migraines, even in people without depression. Tricyclic antidepressants may reduce the frequency of migraines by affecting the level of serotonin and other brain chemicals. Amitriptyline is the only tricyclic antidepressant proved to effectively prevent migraines.

Other tricyclic antidepressants are sometimes used because they may have fewer side effects than amitriptyline. These medications can cause sleepiness, dry mouth, constipation, weight gain and other side effects.

Another class of antidepressants called selective serotonin reuptake inhibitors hasn't been proved to be effective for migraine prevention. These drugs may even worsen or trigger headaches. However, research suggests that one serotonin and norepinephrine reuptake inhibitor, venlafaxine (Effexor XR), may be helpful in preventing migraines.

Anti-seizure drugs. Some anti-seizure drugs, such as topiramate (Topamax) and valproate sodium (Depacon), seem to reduce the frequency of migraines. These anti-seizure drugs may cause side effects.

Valproate sodium may cause nausea, tremor, weight gain, hair loss and dizziness. Valproate sodium products should not be used in pregnant women or women who may become pregnant. Topiramate may cause diarrhea, nausea, weight loss, memory difficulties and concentration problems.

OnabotulinumtoxinA (Botox). OnabotulinumtoxinA (Botox) has been shown to be helpful specifically in treating chronic migraines in adults. Botox is injected into the muscles of the forehead and neck. The treatment usually needs to be repeated every 12 weeks.

Relief is typically experienced within 10 to 14 days, and most will discontinue use if no effect is noted after two to three injections. If effective, the treatment is repeated about every 12 weeks.

Complementary and integrative treatment

Several integrative therapies are used to treat headache pain:

Acupuncture

Acupuncture may help relieve headache pain, but researchers haven't been able to conclude what it is about acupuncture that produces this effect. In one review, researchers studied the results of 22 trials, which included nearly 5,000 people. This literature review showed that at least six sessions of acupuncture helped prevent migraines. Then, a study of 12 trials with around 2,300 participants led researchers to find that acupuncture can effectively treat tension headaches.

However, more high-quality studies are needed before researchers can say with certainty how acupuncture helps treat headaches — and say for certain that acupuncture truly is an effective treatment for headache pain. Learn more about acupuncture starting on page 94.

Biofeedback

Biofeedback is a relaxation technique that uses equipment or devices to teach you how to monitor and control certain physical responses related to stress, such as muscle tension. Many studies of biofeedback and tension headaches have shown that it can be an effective treatment. Likewise, studies have shown that people who use biofeedback have migraines less often.

But more research is needed to prove its effectiveness in both treating and preventing headaches. Learn more about biofeedback starting on page 66.

Massage

Massage therapy may help reduce the frequency of migraines. Researchers continue to study the effectiveness of massage therapy in preventing migraines. Although limited evidence from small studies suggests that massage therapy may be helpful for migraines, there's currently not enough scientific proof available to say whether or not it's an effective treatment. Learn more about massage starting on page 82.

Yoga

Although more research is needed, studies that have been done suggest that yoga may help treat headaches in several ways.

For example, some research shows that practicing yoga for three months reduces how often migraines occur, as well as how intense and painful these headaches are. Researchers reached similar conclusions when studying the effects of a regular yoga practice on tension headache.

Yoga is said to help balance the mind, body and spirit, leading to a calmness that can, in part, decrease tension and improve posture in a way that can help relieve headache pain.

Relaxation exercises

Relaxation exercises help the body respond to stress — as well as pain — more effectively. One type of relaxation exercise, progressive muscle relaxation, is widely used to help manage and prevent headaches. When you're relaxed, you breathe more deeply, and in turn, more oxygen gets to the brain. This seems to prevent headaches. When practiced together with biofeedback, relaxation exercises can cut the number and severity of headaches in half, according to the American Migraine Foundation.

Research into how well relaxation techniques can help treat and prevent headaches is still in its early stages. Many of the findings from studies that have been done are not clear enough for relaxation exercises to be recommended for headaches. Other studies were not of good enough quality.

However, early clinical research shows that relaxation exercises may help make headaches less intense and less frequent. Some research shows that relaxation exercises, when they're practiced twice a week for two weeks, lead to fewer tension headaches and lessen the severity of migraines.

Mindfulness

Although research is still in its early stages, mindfulness has been shown to improve how the body responds to physical pain. The National Center for Complementary and Integrative Health is currently studying the effect of mindfulness meditation on migraines. Learn more about mindfulness meditation on page 57.

Herbs, vitamins and minerals

Several dietary supplements have been studied and are currently under review for use in treating and preventing headaches.

Guidelines from the American Academy of Neurology and the American Headache Society have classified a handful of supplements in terms of their effectiveness in preventing migraines:

- **Effective:** Butterbur
- **Probably effective:** Feverfew, magnesium and riboflavin
- **Possibly effective:** Coenzyme Q10

Although some evidence shows that feverfew and butterbur may prevent migraines or reduce their severity, study results are mixed. Currently, strong research suggests that taking an oral feverfew supplement can help prevent migraines by reducing inflammation and preventing the blood vessels from constricting, both of which can lead to headaches. However, more and better quality studies are needed to confirm effectiveness and safety.

As for butterbur, there's good scientific evidence supporting its use for pain relief and headache prevention. However, because of long-term safety concerns, it isn't recommended for headache treatment or prevention.

Magnesium supplements are useful in preventing migraine, particularly in those who have migraine with aura. In addition, magnesium is one of very few treatments safely used in pregnancy. Finally, many people have low body stores of magnesium, particularly older adults, those on chronic medications or those who drink alcohol regularly. This can make replacing magnesium beneficial.

A high dose of riboflavin (vitamin B-2) also may prevent migraines or reduce the frequency of headaches. Guidelines from the American Academy of Neurology and American Headache Society recommend that riboflavin be considered for migraine prevention.

Additional research suggests that coenzyme Q10 may help prevent and decrease the frequency of migraines. In their guidelines, both the American Academy of Neurology and the American Headache Society recommend that coenzyme Q10 be considered for migraine prevention. As with

other integrative therapies, more good-quality, larger trials are needed to confirm these findings. Learn more about coenzyme Q10 on page 110.

As with all herbs, vitamins and minerals, tell your health care team what you're taking. Even more important, discuss any supplements before you start taking them to ensure that they're safe for you. Learn more about supplements starting on page 102.

Our take

Of all the integrative therapies studied for headache treatment and prevention, feverfew has the most scientific evidence supporting its effectiveness and safety.

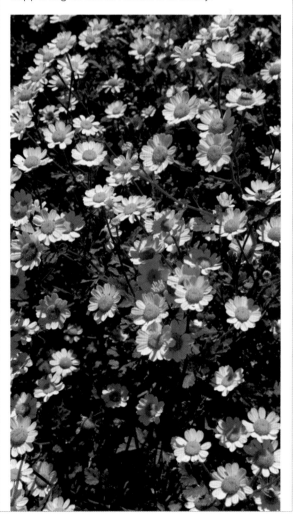

Insomnia

Almost everyone has occasional sleepless nights, perhaps due to stress, heartburn, or drinking too much caffeine or alcohol. Insomnia is a lack of sleep that occurs on a regular or frequent basis, and often for no apparent reason.

How much sleep is enough varies from person to person. Although most adults need seven to nine hours of sleep, this is an average — how much you need may vary. You may do well on less sleep, or you may need more.

Insomnia can affect not only your energy level and mood, but also your health because sleep helps bolster your immune system. Without enough sleep, you may get sick more often. Fatigue, at any age, leads to diminished mental alertness and concentration. Lack of sleep caused by insomnia is linked to accidents both on the road and on the job.

Insomnia may be either temporary or chronic. But you don't necessarily have to live with the sleepless nights of insomnia. Some simple changes in your daily routine and habits may result in better sleep.

Conventional treatment

No matter what your age, insomnia usually is treatable. The key often lies in changes to your routine during the day and when you go to bed.

Sleep hygiene

Key coping skills that can help overcome sleep problems include:
- Sticking to a sleep schedule
- Avoiding "trying" to sleep
- Hiding the bedroom clocks
- Exercising and staying active
- Avoiding or limiting caffeine, alcohol and nicotine
- Checking your medications for drugs that may affect sleep
- Dealing with painful health conditions
- Finding ways to relax
- Avoiding or limiting naps

Medication

If sleep hygiene measures don't work or you believe that another condition, such as depression, restless legs syndrome or anxiety, is causing your insomnia, talk to your doctor. He or she may recommend that you take medications to promote relaxation or sleep.

Several medications, both over-the-counter and prescription, are available — and each has pros and cons that are important to weigh with your health care team.

Nonprescription medications. Nonprescription sleep aids contain antihistamines to induce drowsiness. They're OK for occasional sleepless nights, but they, too, often lose their effectiveness the more you take them and are not recommended for long-term use. Antihistamines also may cause daytime sleepiness, dizziness, confusion, cognitive decline and difficulty emptying your bladder completely (urinary retention).

Many sleeping pills contain diphenhydramine and doxylamine, which aren't recommended for people who have certain conditions, such as closed-angle glaucoma, asthma, chronic obstructive pulmonary disease or severe liver disease.

Prescription medications. Taking prescription sleeping pills, such as zolpidem (Ambien, Intermezzo, others), eszopiclone (Lunesta), zaleplon (Sonata) or ramelteon (Rozerem), for a couple of weeks until there's less stress in your life may help you get to sleep until you notice benefits from behavioral self-help measures. The antidepressants trazodone and mirtazapine (Remeron) also may help with insomnia.

Doctors generally don't recommend prescription sleeping pills for more than a few weeks because they may cause unwanted side effects. Prescription sleeping pills can cause daytime grogginess and increase the risk of falling. In addition, they can be habit-forming. Talk to your health care team about these medications and other possible side effects they may cause. Plus, keep in mind that your goal is to develop the ability to sleep without the help of medication.

Complementary and integrative treatment

Many integrative treatments are used for insomnia, and several may offer some benefit.

Melatonin

Melatonin is an over-the-counter supplement that's marketed as a way to help overcome insomnia. It's generally considered safe to use melatonin for a few weeks, but the safety of long-term use is unknown.

In terms of research, no convincing evidence exists to prove that melatonin is an effective treatment for insomnia. Learn more about melatonin on page 109.

Valerian

This dietary supplement is sold as a sleep aid because it has a mildly sedating effect, although it hasn't been well-studied.

Discuss valerian with your doctor before trying it. Some people who have used high doses or used it long term may have had liver damage, although it's not clear if valerian caused the damage. Learn more about valerian on page 121.

Relaxation exercises

Relaxation techniques can be helpful as part of overall sleep hygiene and as treatment for chronic insomnia. Progressive muscle relaxation may help with nighttime anxiety, and mindfulness-based stress reduction appears to be as effective as prescription sleep medication. Learn more about relaxation exercises on page 43.

Meditation

Several small studies suggest that meditation, along with conventional treatment, may help improve sleep and reduce stress. Learn more about meditation starting on page 56.

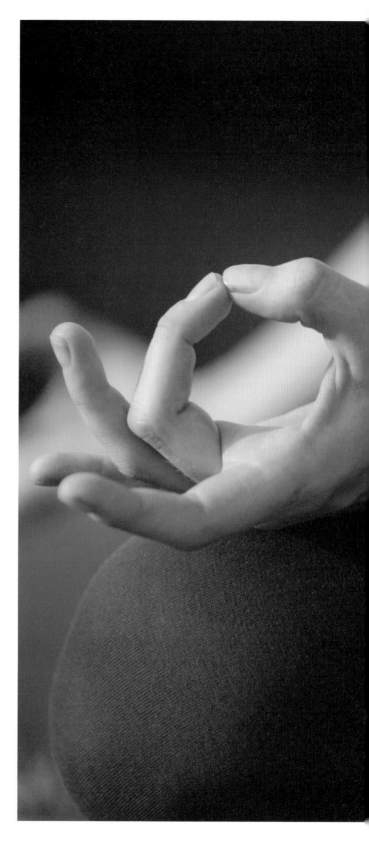

Yoga or tai chi

Some studies suggest that a regular practice of yoga or tai chi can help improve sleep quality. Learn about yoga and tai chi on page 29.

Acupuncture

There's some evidence that acupuncture may be beneficial for people with insomnia, but more research is needed. If you choose to try acupuncture along with your conventional treatment, ask your doctor how to find a qualified practitioner. Learn about acupuncture starting on page 94.

Hypnosis

Hypnosis uses the power of suggestion to help individuals overcome various health issues, such as insomnia. Several early studies report that hypnosis may decrease the amount of time it takes to fall asleep, increase the duration of sleep, and improve sleep quality. However, this research is not well-designed or reported and cannot be considered definitive. Learn more about hypnosis starting on page 69.

May help and likely won't hurt

Although research is unclear about the value of these therapies for insomnia, the risk of trying them is relatively low:

Aromatherapy. Aromatherapy uses essential oils from plants with the intention of preventing or treating illness, reducing stress or enhancing well-being. Diluted oils are applied to the skin, sprayed in the air or inhaled. Early research suggests that chamomile or lavender aromatherapy may be beneficial for improving sleep quality. Learn more about aromatherapy on page 90.

Music therapy. Music is used to influence physical, emotional, cognitive and social well-being, and improve quality of life for healthy people, as well as those who are disabled or ill. Music therapy involves either listening to or performing music with a certified music therapist for a therapeutic goal. In older adults, music therapy may help improve sleep quality and duration, as well as shorten the time needed to fall asleep, among other benefits. Music therapy is generally known to be safe, and there's good scientific evidence that it can help treat insomnia. Learn more about music therapy on page 50.

Our take

Of all the research that's been done on integrative techniques for insomnia, melatonin and music therapy are shown to be the most effective in treating sleeplessness. However, clinical experience at Mayo Clinic shows that a mind-body practice can aid stress management while helping prepare the brain for sleep, especially when that mind-body practice is included as part of a bedtime ritual. Practicing guided imagery 30 minutes before bedtime, for example, has been shown to be a beneficial way to treat insomnia.

Don't ignore sleep problems

When it comes to your health, sleep is as important as a healthy diet and regular exercise. Whatever your reason for sleep loss, insomnia can impact you both mentally and physically.

The impact can be cumulative. People with chronic insomnia are more likely than others to develop psychiatric problems such as depression and anxiety disorders. Long-term sleep deprivation can also increase the severity of chronic diseases, such as high blood pressure and heart disease.

And it's clear that insufficient sleep can lead to serious or even fatal accidents. According to the National Highway Traffic Safety Administration, driver fatigue causes more than 100,000 crashes each year.

Irritable bowel syndrome

Irritable bowel syndrome (IBS) is one of the most common gastrointestinal disorders. Yet it's also one that many people aren't comfortable talking about. Irritable bowel syndrome is characterized by abdominal pain or cramping and changes in bowel function — including bloating, gas, diarrhea and constipation — problems most people don't like to discuss.

IBS affects between 25 million and 45 million people in the United States. Irritable bowel syndrome is the sixth-leading condition that doctors make. The disorder accounts for between 2.4 million and 3.5 million doctor visits a year.

For most people, signs and symptoms of irritable bowel syndrome are mild. Only a small percentage of people have severe signs and symptoms.

Fortunately, unlike more serious intestinal diseases such as ulcerative colitis and Crohn's disease, irritable bowel syndrome doesn't cause inflammation or changes in bowel tissue or increase your risk of colorectal cancer. In many cases, it's possible to control the symptoms of irritable bowel syndrome by managing your diet, lifestyle and stress.

Conventional treatment

Because it's still not clear what causes irritable bowel syndrome, treatment focuses on the relief of symptoms so that you can live your life as fully and normally as possible. In most cases, you can successfully control mild symptoms of irritable bowel syndrome by learning to manage stress and making changes in your diet and lifestyle.

But if your problems are moderate or severe, you may need more help than lifestyle changes alone can offer. Your doctor may suggest:

Fiber supplements

Taking fiber supplements such as psyllium (Metamucil, Konsyl, others) or methylcellulose (Citrucel) with fluids may help control the symptom of constipation in irritable bowel syndrome.

Anti-diarrheal medications

Over-the-counter medications such as loperamide (Imodium A-D) can help control diarrhea.

Changes in diet

Eating smaller meals more often and eating smaller portions are two dietary changes you can make that may help relieve IBS symptoms. Choosing foods that are low in fat and high in carbohydrates, such as pasta, rice, whole-grain breads and cereals, fruits, and vegetables, also may help.

Finally, you may have heard of FODMAPs, which stands for **f**ermentable, **o**ligosaccharides, **d**isaccharides, **m**onosaccharides and **p**olyols. The FODMAP diet involves eating less or avoiding foods containing carbohydrates that are hard for your body to digest — foods in each of these categories. Certain fruits, vegetables, dairy products, wheat and rye products, honey, foods that contain high-fructose corn syrup, and products that contain certain sweeteners are all featured on the low-FODMAP list. Learn more about this diet and how it can help manage IBS symptoms on the next page.

Anticholinergic medications

Some people need drugs that affect certain activities of the nervous system (anticholinergics) to relieve painful bowel spasms.

Antidepressant medications

In addition to improving mood, antidepressants can relieve pain, so they're sometimes prescribed for irritable bowel syndrome. Tricyclic antidepressants have a tendency to slow down how quickly food moves through the intestines, which can be helpful for IBS with diarrhea — however, these antidepressants have side effects and should be used with care for those who have constipation.

More on FODMAPs

FODMAP stands for:

Fermentable
Oligosaccharides (fructans and galactans, found in wheat, garlic, and dried beans and peas)
Disaccharides (lactose, found in dairy products such as milk)
Monosaccharides (excess fructose, including honey and some fruits)
And
Polyols (sugar alcohols such as sorbitol, maltitol, mannitol, xylitol and isomalt and other low-calorie sweeteners)

The body doesn't absorb the sugars and carbohydrates in the foods found in these categories well. This, in turn, can lead to bloating and gas production.

A diet that's low in these foods can help reduce the amount of gas your body produces. This type of diet is often used to help treat a variety of digestive issues, including diarrhea and constipation. That makes this diet helpful for conditions such as irritable bowel syndrome.

The low-FODMAP diet has been accepted by Australia's Therapeutic Guidelines as a primary therapy for managing symptoms of irritable bowel syndrome. The low-FODMAP diet can be modified to meet a person's specific needs and preferences.

Once you have discussed a low-FODMAP diet with your health care team and decided that it's a good approach for you, generally the first step is to avoid all high-FODMAP foods for four weeks. After four weeks, you can start to reintroduce the foods you eliminated back into your diet. The ultimate goal is to include as many of them as possible, as long as they're not causing symptoms.

Most people start to notice improvements in their symptoms in a few days, but it generally takes a few weeks to get the most benefit from this dietary change.

Your health care team will guide you on how you should specifically follow the low-FODMAP diet, including how many servings of which types of foods are best for you.

Counseling

If antidepressant medications don't help, you may have better results from counseling if stress tends to exacerbate your symptoms.

Medications specifically for IBS

Two drugs are available to treat IBS: alosetron (Lotronex) and lubiprostone (Amitiza).

Alosetron (Lotronex). This nerve receptor antagonist is supposed to relax the colon and slow the movement of waste through the lower bowel. But the drug was removed from the market just nine months after its approval when it was linked to serious, life-threatening effects. In 2002, the Food and Drug Administration (FDA) decided to allow alosetron to be sold again — with restrictions. The drug can be prescribed only by doctors enrolled in a special program and is intended for severe cases of diarrhea-predominant IBS in women who don't respond to other treatments. It isn't approved for men.

Lubiprostone (Amitiza). This drug works by increasing fluid secretion in your small intestine to help with the passage of stool. It is approved for women age 18 and older who have IBS with constipation. Its effectiveness in men is not proved, nor is its long-term safety.

Common side effects include nausea, diarrhea and abdominal pain. Lubiprostone is generally prescribed only for women with IBS and severe constipation for whom other treatments haven't been successful.

Complementary and integrative treatment

The following integrative therapies may help relieve symptoms of irritable bowel syndrome:

Probiotics

Probiotics are "good" bacteria that are found naturally in your intestines. They're also found in some foods, such as yogurt, and are available in dietary supplements, such as capsules, tablets and powders. Probiotics may be able to help improve the health of your "gut microbiome" — the environment in your digestive system where bacteria live. The bacteria in your digestive system are an essential part of your immune system. When your gut microbiome is in good shape, so is the rest of your body. Probiotics help your digestive system function well, which, in turn, helps your entire body perform at its best.

Many varieties and combinations of probiotics have been studied for their possible use in treating irritable bowel syndrome. Current research shows that taking probiotics can help reduce symptoms of irritable bowel syndrome, including pain, flatulence, bloating and stool frequency. It may also help reduce inflammation. However, not all studies have had positive results, and if taken in large doses, probiotics may cause diarrhea. Learn more about probiotics on page 108.

Peppermint oil

When used as a dietary supplement, peppermint helps treat IBS, among other digestive problems and medical conditions. It has been studied most extensively for irritable bowel syndrome. Studies show that it can improve IBS-related symptoms such as cramping and bloating. However, more research is needed, and peppermint supplements can cause adverse effects in some people.

Fennel

Fennel seeds have been used as herbal medicines in Europe and China for centuries, and fennel tea is often used to treat digestive problems. It may help relieve symptoms of IBS, as well, but more research is needed.

Hypnosis

Early research of hypnosis suggests that it may help treat irritable bowel syndrome, but better studies are needed. Learn more about hypnotherapy on page 69.

Our take

Of all the integrative medicine techniques studied for treating irritable bowel syndrome, fennel, hypnotherapy, peppermint oil and probiotics show the most promise, with the strongest scientific evidence supporting their use. But therapies that have fewer studies may still be worth considering if these aren't helping. Acupuncture, for example, is successful in treating IBS in many cases and is another illustration of why it's important to discuss all of your options for treating a chronic condition with your health care team.

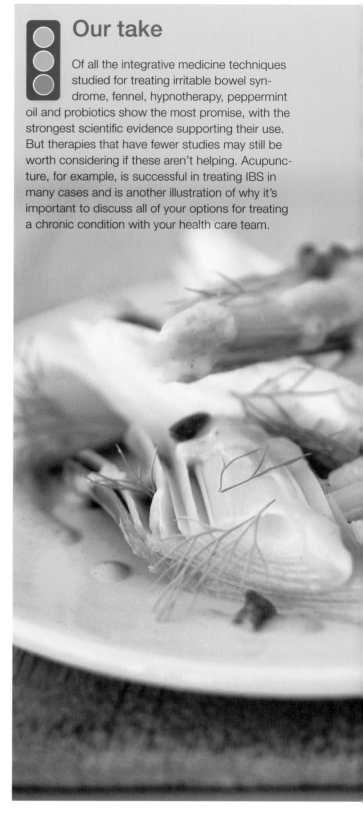

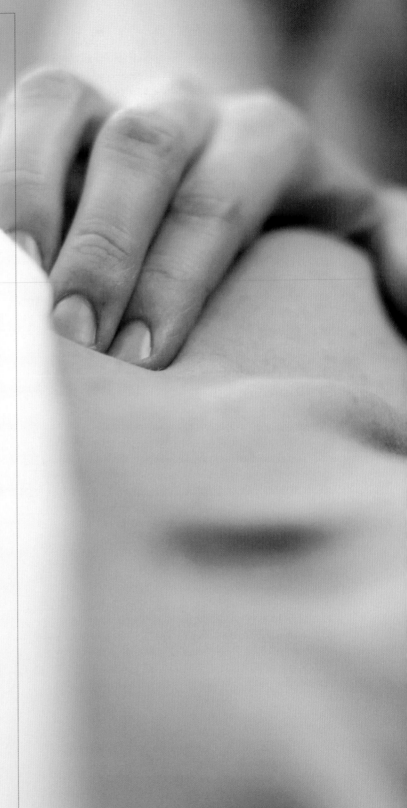

Dealing with stress may prevent IBS

Finding ways to deal with stress can be helpful in preventing or alleviating symptoms of IBS. Stress management strategies include:

Counseling. Sometimes, a health care professional such as a psychologist or psychiatrist can help you learn how to reduce stress. Cognitive behavioral therapy, which can help you modify thoughts and behaviors; working on your relationships with others; and various forms of relaxation and stress management are all ways that counseling can help. Various forms of counseling can help relieve anxiety and other mental health issues, as well as reduce symptoms of IBS.

Biofeedback. This stress-reduction technique helps you reduce muscle tension and slow your heart rate with the feedback help of a device. You're then taught how to produce these changes yourself. Learn more about how biofeedback is used for stress management starting on page 66.

Regular exercise, yoga, massage or meditation. You can take classes in yoga and meditation or practice the therapies at home using books or tapes. Learn more about yoga on page 29, massage starting on page 82, and meditation starting on page 56.

Progressive relaxation exercises. Start by tightening the muscles in your feet, then concentrate on slowly letting all of the tension go. Next, tighten and relax your calves. Continue until the muscles in your body, including those in your eyes and scalp, are completely relaxed. Learn more about progressive muscle relaxation exercises starting on page 44.

Deep breathing. Most adults breathe from their chests. But you become calmer when you breathe from your diaphragm, the muscle that separates your chest from your abdomen. When you inhale, allow your belly to expand with air; when you exhale, your belly contracts. Learn more about deep breathing starting on page 46.

Hypnosis. A trained professional teaches you how to relax and then guides you as you imagine your intestinal muscles becoming smooth and calm. Learn more about hypnosis on page 69.

Stress and mood disorders

Modern life is full of pressures, fears and frustration. In other words, it's stressful. Racing against deadlines, sitting in traffic, arguing with your spouse — all of these situations make your body react as if you were facing a physical threat.

This reaction, called the fight-or-flight response, gave early humans the energy to fight aggressors or run from predators. Today, instead of offering protection, your body's stress response may actually make you *more* vulnerable to stress-related health problems if it's constantly activated.

It's normal to feel anxious or worried at times. Everyone does. But if you often feel anxious without reason and your worries disrupt your daily life, you may have what's called generalized anxiety disorder. This condition causes excessive or unrealistic anxiety and worry about life circumstances, usually without a readily identifiable cause.

Fortunately, there's help for chronic stress and anxiety. Treatment ranges from learning new coping skills to professional counseling or therapy. Several complementary and integrative therapies may also prove helpful in easing your emotional and physical burden.

Conventional treatment

If you're under continuous stress that appears to have no end in sight, you may be able to help yourself by implementing some key changes in your life. Professional counseling also can help. A buildup of stress can worsen generalized anxiety disorder, in which case a combination of medications and psychotherapy is often recommended.

Self-care

There are three fundamental ways in which to manage stress: by changing your environment so that daily demands aren't so high, by learning how to better cope with the demands in your environment, or by doing both.

Techniques that can help you manage stress include identifying and addressing the problems you can change, letting go of stressors beyond your control, taking good care of yourself, maintaining a healthy diet, exercising and finding time for relaxation, and relying on certain people to help you through the rough spots.

Aside from self-care, several types of medications and therapies are used to help treat stress and mood disorders.

Medications

Medications that are commonly used to help treat stress and mood disorders include:

Anti-anxiety drugs. Benzodiazepines are sedatives that often ease anxiety within 30 to 90 minutes. Because they can be habit-forming, your doctor may prescribe them for only a short time to help you get through a particularly anxious period. Side effects include unsteadiness, drowsiness, reduced muscle coordination and problems with balance. These medications can also cause memory problems.

Antidepressants. These drugs influence the activity of certain brain chemicals (neurotransmitters) to help nerve cells (neurons) in your brain send and receive messages. It may take several weeks before you notice the antidepressants' full effects. You may need to try more than one to find which drug works best for you. Antidepressants are used to help relieve symptoms of depression as well as treat anxiety disorders.

Psychotherapy

A common form of psychotherapy used to treat anxiety is cognitive behavioral therapy. During treatment sessions, a therapist helps you identify distorted thoughts and beliefs that trigger psychological stress, fear or depression. Through psychotherapy, you learn to replace negative thoughts with more positive, realistic perceptions, and you learn ways to view and cope with life events differently.

Complementary and integrative treatment

Various forms of integrative therapies are used to treat stress and anxiety. The success of these treatments often depends on each individual's response. With the exception of some herbal therapies, most are relatively safe and have few side effects.

Music therapy

Whether it's live or recorded, classical or another style, music therapy is generally a safe mind-body technique that has been shown to be helpful in treating stress and anxiety, depression, and a variety of other mood disorders.

Music helps produce a relaxation response in your body that leads to a lower heart rate, lower blood pressure, less tension, and lower levels of stress hormones in your body. Learn more about music therapy starting on page 50.

Art therapy

Various forms of art therapy can help you work through your feelings, which can help you cope with stress and anxiety. Learn more about art therapy starting on page 48.

Hypnotherapy

A trancelike state in which you become more focused and aware and open to suggestion, hypnotherapy has been shown to be an effective treatment for a variety of conditions, including anxiety and post-traumatic stress disorder. Hypnotherapy should be used cautiously with mental illnesses. Learn more about hypnotherapy starting on page 69.

Yoga

A combination of relaxation and exercise, yoga can be an effective way to reduce stress and anxiety and help treat a variety of mental health conditions. Although it's generally considered to be safe, yoga may pose risks for some people. Learn more about yoga on page 29.

Meditation

Researchers studying meditation have found that it can help reduce the effects of stress and can help treat depression. However, meditation should be used with caution with underlying mental health conditions. Learn more about meditation starting on page 56.

Relaxation therapy

Relaxation therapy encompasses numerous techniques ranging from paced respiration and deep breathing to meditation and progressive muscle relaxation. Most types of relaxation therapy involve repetition of a single word, phrase or muscular activity and promote "emptying" your mind of external thoughts and stressors. Learn more about different types of relaxation therapies starting on page 43.

Biofeedback

For this technique, a practitioner measures your body's physiological response to stress or anxiety, which is displayed to you as auditory or visual signals. By increasing your awareness of your body's responses, you attempt to counter the signals with relaxation methods. Biofeedback is used for stress and depression, although more research is needed to prove its effectiveness. Learn more about biofeedback starting on page 66.

Massage

A number of studies indicate that massage can help reduce stress and anxiety symptoms and help treat other mental health conditions. Research also shows that massage may help reduce depression. Learn more about massage starting on page 82.

Aromatherapy

Research on the effectiveness of aromatherapy — the therapeutic use of essential oils extracted from plants — is limited. However, some studies have shown that it might have health benefits, including relief from anxiety and depression. Learn more about aromatherapy on page 90.

Dietary supplements

St. John's wort, SAMe, omega-3 fatty acids, 5-HTP and valerian are some of the most common supplements used for anxiety and depression.

St. John's wort isn't approved by the Food and Drug Administration to treat depression in the United States, but it is a popular depression treatment in Europe. Although it may help treat anxiety and mild or moderate depression, it can interact with many different medications and supplements, so be sure to talk with your doctor before taking this supplement. Learn more about St. John's wort on page 119.

Like St. John's wort, SAMe isn't approved by the Food and Drug Administration to treat depression in the U.S., but it's popular in Europe for treating depression. SAMe may be helpful, but more research is needed. SAMe may trigger mania in people with bipolar disorder.

Omega-3 fatty acids are healthy fats found in cold-water fish, flaxseed, walnuts and some other foods. Some research shows that omega-3 supplements may help treat depression. While considered generally safe, omega-3 supplements may interact with other medications. Although eating foods with omega-3 fatty acids appears to have heart-healthy benefits, more research is needed to determine if it has an effect on preventing or improving depression. Learn more about omega-3 fatty acids on page 106.

The supplement called 5-hydroxytryptophan (5-HTP) is available over-the-counter in the U.S., but requires a prescription in some countries. The use of 5-HTP may play a role in improving serotonin levels, a chemical that affects mood — but evidence is only preliminary and more research is needed.

Valerian has been studied for treating anxiety, but research detailing its effectiveness isn't strong for either. Some people who have taken valerian reported less stress and anxiety, but others did not. Learn more about valerian on page 121.

Our take

Among the most promising integrative therapies for relieving stress and symptoms of mood disorders, there is good support for counseling, art and music therapy, as well as yoga for both anxiety and depression. Meditation and relaxation therapies are effective ways to manage anxiety. St. John's wort and hypnotherapy have strong support for their use in treating depression with some cautions.

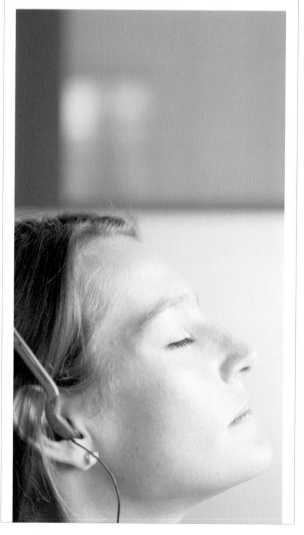

The brain-body connection

A visit with Dr. Fleming

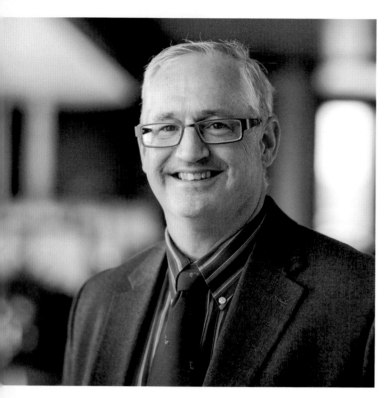

Kevin C. Fleming, M.D.
General Internal Medicine
Mayo Clinic

Dr. Fleming is the director of the Fibromyalgia and Chronic Fatigue Clinic at Mayo Clinic, Rochester, Minnesota.

Earlier in this book, you read about mind-body medicine and how the mind and body are connected. In this section, we'll take this idea a step further and look at how your brain works — and how it can affect several different conditions. Fibromyalgia, chronic fatigue, irritable bowel syndrome and chronic daily headaches are examples.

These conditions may sound familiar to you, or you or a loved one may be coping with one or more of them. These are just a few conditions that have many signs and symptoms in common, such as muscle pain, fatigue, sleep disorders and depression.

But what these conditions also have in common is that often, doctors can't find a cause for, or a way to treat, their symptoms.

Researchers and medical experts think that a concept called *central sensitization* may be the cause behind symptoms and syndromes that don't appear to have a physical cause. This is where the mind-body connection comes in.

Integrative therapies such as the ones you're learning about in this book can help relieve symptoms related to central sensitization — and have been used for years in Mayo Clinic's pain rehabilitation programs. Researchers are finding that an array of integrative techniques can help reduce the pain and other symptoms of these disorders. Many of these therapies and techniques strengthen the mind-body connection and can help you rewire your brain in a way that can help "turn down" the nerve signaling in your brain that may be causing certain signs and symptoms.

In fact, integrative therapies are becoming an increasingly integral component of treating these painful disorders now that medication is largely shown to be unhelpful and even harmful in some cases. You'll learn more about which therapies are helpful later in this section. For now, let's start off with a basic understanding of what central sensitization is and how it works in your body.

The brain-body connection

Many medical conditions in today's world lack a physical cause or a rational explanation of what's going on the body.

Test after test and exam after exam often lead nowhere, except to frustration and disappointment for those who are coping with symptoms that they don't understand and don't know how to manage. Frustration mounts when doctor after doctor can't provide answers or name a specific condition that's causing the symptoms.

Years of research have been spent on this scenario, and today, medical experts believe they have an answer to what causes symptoms and syndromes that don't appear to have a physical cause: *central sensitization*.

What it is

Put simply, central sensitization describes changes in your nervous system that make you hypersensitive to pain.

Central sensitization causes a variety of symptoms to occur in the body. Because they're so varied, symptoms are hard to piece together, and it can be difficult to understand that it's all one disorder. Central sensitization is related to most types of chronic pain.

In central sensitization, symptoms and syndromes occur because of a bad circuit (or bad circuits) in the central nervous system. Nerves become rewired, leading your brain to believe that ordinary sensations, such as touch, are harmful or painful.

How it works

Tiny sensor cells cover every square inch of your body. The exceptions to this are your hair and fingernails. That's why you can generally cut them without experiencing too much, if any, pain. Sensors are present in the skin, gut, muscles, joints, bones, balance system, nerves, vascular system and vision system. Additional sensors help you hear, taste and smell.

Typically, these sensors monitor your environment and send a variety of physical sensations to the brain, keeping track of sounds, sights, tastes, pain and other reactions to stimuli.

Many different nerve cells help get information from these sensors to the spinal cord and to different areas of the brain, much like how information travels along a phone line. From there, the brain interprets the information and tells your body how to deal with it. For example, if you're too hot, you may go somewhere to cool off. If you're thirsty, you may drink some water. These are examples of how signals are sent to the brain, which then informs you how to respond. This can happen anywhere in the body.

In central sensitization, the signal sent to your spinal cord and brain is strengthened or, put another way, turned up. It's similar to turning up the volume on a radio. When you turn up the volume, the music gets louder — this is similar to what happens when the signals to your spinal cord and brain are strengthened.

However, unlike the volume on your radio, in central sensitization, once these signals are turned up, all of your sensors are on overdrive. Sounds can seem louder, lights can seem brighter, movement can hurt more and the digestive system may encounter more problems. The idea behind central sensitization is that this "upregulation" is what's causing symptoms to become more bothersome and more difficult to treat — or to understand why they're happening altogether.

In central sensitization, normal messages from the nerve endings in your body are magnified by the time they reach the thinking part of your brain. Research using functional magnetic resonance imaging (fMRI) of the brain has shown that during central sensitization, you can actually see changes in how the brain routes and processes messages. When the brain receives messages from the sensors in your body, it thinks that there's a disaster happening, even though almost nothing is happening at all.

Current research has linked central sensitization to a number of previously mysterious and pain-related conditions, such as:

- Peripheral neuropathy
- Arthritis
- Migraine
- Fibromyalgia
- Irritable bowel syndrome
- Temporomandibular joint disorder (TMD)

Several other conditions you may have heard of also seem to be linked to central sensitization. They include:

- Chronic fatigue syndrome
- Systemic exertion intolerance disease (SEID)
- Postural orthostatic tachycardia syndrome
- Complex regional pain syndrome

Other forms of chronic pain, such as interstitial cystitis or atypical facial pain, show a modest link to central sensitization, as well. And finally, there's suspicion — but not much evidence yet — that other conditions, such as restless legs syndrome or post-traumatic stress disorder, may also involve central sensitization.

Symptoms

A "turned up" central nervous system leads to a range of symptoms that become worse over time. In a study published in the journal *Pain Practice*, researchers came up with a central sensitization inventory that measures 25 different symptoms linked to central sensitization and can help health care providers determine if their patients are experiencing this disorder.

At Mayo Clinic, Arya B. Mohabbat, M.D., and other Mayo Clinic physicians and researchers created a similar list of symptoms. Here's more on each of them.

Pain

About half of the symptoms of central sensitization fall into the broad category of pain. These

David's story

A man in his 50s, David came to Mayo Clinic because he was experiencing a variety of symptoms – but none of his doctors could find a cause for them.

When he arrived at Mayo Clinic, David was assigned to a doctor with whom he discussed his symptoms. Among them, David was fatigued and was experiencing muscle pain, joint pain, neck stiffness, tingling sensations, pain in his jaw and lightheadedness. He also said that mentally, he felt foggy and confused.

After hearing about all of David's symptoms, his doctor wondered if he might be experiencing central sensitization. She ordered several tests to rule out other causes for his symptoms, and one by one, they learned that there were no other possible causes for his symptoms.

Based on what his tests ruled out, in combination with various exams from the specialists he saw, David's primary Mayo Clinic doctor concluded that David had fibromyalgia – and possibly central sensitization.

David's doctor talked to him about ways they could treat both his fibromyalgia and central sensitization. Low-impact exercise, behavioral changes, stress management, and treatment for any underlying depression or anxiety would be key. She then referred him to the Mayo Clinic Fibromyalgia Treatment Program.

David struggled to understand what central sensitization was, as well as what was going on in his body and in his mind. He felt as though he was either very sick or losing his mind. It was hard for him to understand how something happening in his central nervous system could be causing so many varied and unrelated symptoms. But in essence, that's what was happening. That's what central sensitization is.

Over time, David learned how to manage his many symptoms through the techniques you'll read about later in this section.

Although David couldn't eradicate all of his symptoms, he was able to manage them well enough that he could go back to living his life in a way that was both productive and enjoyable.

symptoms include *myalgia* and *arthralgia* — in other words, muscle and joint pain that don't appear to be caused by inflammation.

Numbness or tingling

Some people who are experiencing central sensitization say they feel numbness or tingling sensations. Medically, these sensations are known as *paresthesia*. You may have numbness or tingling sensations in place of pain, or along with pain.

Headaches

Headaches are sometimes a symptom of central sensitization. They may be tension headaches or migraine headaches.

Temporomandibular joint (TMJ) dysfunction

Temporomandibular joint (TMJ) dysfunction is another possible symptom of central sensitization. TMJ dysfunction involves pain in the jaw joint and in the muscles that control jaw movement. As is the case with other symptoms, pain is there, but there's no jaw injury to explain it.

Irritable bowel syndrome (IBS)

People with central sensitization often report symptoms of irritable bowel syndrome (IBS). Irritable bowel syndrome affects the large intestine (colon). It commonly causes cramping, abdominal pain, bloating, gas, diarrhea and constipation.

Interstitial cystitis

Bladder pressure, bladder pain, the urge to void frequently and sometimes pelvic pain are all symptoms of interstitial cystitis — and can all be symptoms of central sensitization. When people have symptoms such as these but have no tissue damage or infection, interstitial cystitis is typically the diagnosis.

Chronic pelvic pain

Central sensitization can cause chronic pelvic pain, or pain below the bellybutton. In women, this sometimes goes hand in hand with menstrual problems, so it's important to talk to a gynecologist to eliminate other causes for this kind of pain.

Restless legs syndrome

Restless legs syndrome also often accompanies central sensitization. Symptoms can range from mildly irritating to excruciating. The symptoms tend to get worse in the evening, which can lead to poor sleep and daytime fatigue.

Fatigue

Fatigue is one of the most common symptoms of central sensitization. Often, it's the symptom that brings people to the doctor in the first place. Fatigue is usually present every day, all day, and is no better after sleep. Fatigue is considered chronic if it's present for six months or longer and isn't caused by an underlying medical issue.

Sleep problems

Many people have problems with sleep, whether or not they have restless legs syndrome. They may sleep too much, or they may be unable to sleep at all. Or, they may feel that their sleep is unrefreshing. If you snore a lot, or are overweight, it's best to eliminate sleep apnea as a cause first.

Dizziness and lightheadedness

Central sensitization can lead to feelings of dizziness and lightheadedness. These sensations may happen all the time, or just when someone sits or stands too quickly.

Weakness

Some people who are affected by central sensitization feel a general sense of weakness.

Brain fog

Many people who experience central sensitization say they feel foggy mentally. They say their memory is going, or their attention span is poor or they're just getting dumber. Some will blame this on lack of sleep, but even people who don't have problems sleeping may experience brain fog as part of central sensitization.

Depression and anxiety

Mood disorders is a sensitive topic in central sensitization. For many years, doctors felt that people who reported symptoms such as those listed here were hypochondriacs if there didn't seem to be a cause for their patients' symptoms. In essence, doctors thought that their patients were experiencing a psychological issue when they were, in fact, truly experiencing the symptoms they reported.

Today, medical professionals understand that depression and anxiety can actually be symptoms of central sensitization and that forms of depression or anxiety can actually lead to physical symptoms. Sometimes the burden of chronic physical symptoms can cause mood disorders. No matter what causes depression and anxiety, these are conditions that can be effectively treated.

Sensitivities

Central sensitization can cause symptoms defined as *global sensory hyperresponsiveness*. This means that the body seems to overreact to stimuli, whether it's food, medication or something in the environment. A true allergic reaction may or may not be involved.

Sensitivity to light, loud noises or changes in the weather that others may not notice are other sensitivities that someone with central sensitization may experience.

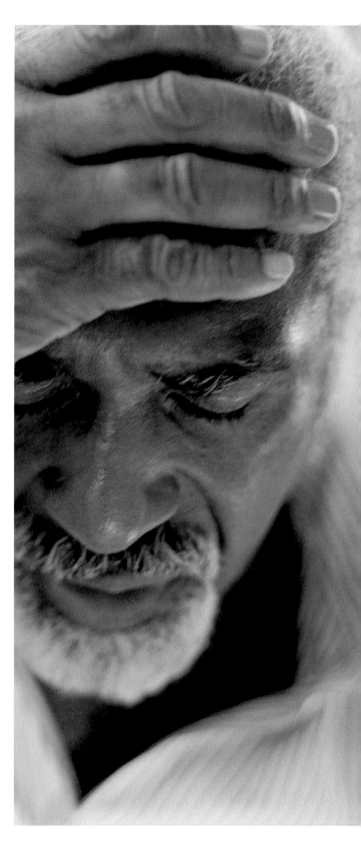

As the sensitivity in the nervous system increases and symptoms get worse and possibly increase in number, it's common for people to become more desperate for relief, and more confused about what's happening in their bodies.

Causes

Central sensitization can be difficult to diagnose, so as you may imagine, finding a cause for central sensitization can also be a challenge.

A mix of factors seems to be behind central sensitization. Unlike other medical conditions and syndromes, there's no one set of causes for central sensitization. However, research has identified more than a dozen different factors that can play a role. Several of these factors may be found in any given person.

Here's what researchers and health care professionals know today about the many causes that may be involved in central sensitization.

A triggering event

One single event can trigger central sensitization and bring symptoms to the forefront.

A serious infection is one example. Some people may say that they got sick, perhaps with a viral infection such as mononucleosis, and never felt like they got better. A chemical exposure or a trauma can lead to central sensitization as well. A car accident, a surgery, or a rheumatic disorder, such as lupus or rheumatoid arthritis, can put strain on the body and ultimately trigger central sensitization. These are all examples of triggers.

Stress

While physical stress has been shown to cause central sensitization, researchers have found that psychological stress or trauma can trigger central sensitization, as well.

These traumas may be sudden and brief, or they may last a few weeks, months or years. Trauma that lasts for a period of time — such as combat service — is known as a prolonged stressor.

Environment

Similar to stress, certain environmental factors may play a role in triggering central sensitization, as well. Researchers count trauma in early life — such as child abuse — certain infections, and emotional stress among environmental factors that can lead to central sensitization.

Mood disorders

Underlying mood disorders can be either a cause or a symptom of central sensitization.

Sleep

Getting enough good-quality sleep is important for physical and psychological health, in general. Although sleep disturbances affect many people for many different reasons, research shows that not getting enough good-quality sleep — in particular, sleep disturbances — can lead to central sensitization.

Sensitivities

You learned earlier in this section that global sensory hyperresponsiveness — the body's overreaction to a stimulus — can be a symptom of central sensitization. However, it can also cause central sensitization.

Changes in other parts of your nervous system

To this point, you've learned that central sensitization is a syndrome that involves your central nervous system — specifically, your brain and your spinal cord. However, another part of your nervous system may play a role in causing this condition, as well.

Your peripheral nervous system links your brain and spinal cord to the other parts of your body, such as your muscles and your skin. Your peripheral nerves are the link from your brain and spinal cord to your muscles and your organs. If these nerves are damaged, communication to and from the brain and spinal cord may be affected.

Chemical changes in your nervous system can also lead to central sensitization. *Neurochemical alterations* and *immunomodulation* are two examples. Put simply, the levels of chemicals involved in sending signals to your brain may be too high or too low.

Your nervous system also helps set the levels of hormones in your system; this level may also be too high or too low, which can lead to changes that cause central sensitization.

Neuroplasticity

Your nervous system changes and adapts throughout your life. This concept is known as *neuroplasticity* — you learned about it earlier in this book. Neuroplasticity is how you learn, change and adapt over time.

Neuroplasticity is also responsible for sending signals to your brain about pain, leading your brain to tell the rest of your body how to respond to it. Similar to the operating system for your computer, neuroplasticity is the operating system for your nervous system.

Most of the time, neuroplasticity is a good thing. However, in central sensitization, your nervous system adapts in ways that aren't helpful.

When the nerves in your peripheral nervous system sense pain, they send information to your brain, which decides how your body should respond to it. Once your body responds to the pain, that's usually the end of the story. But in some people, the pain signals sent to the brain never resolve themselves. That's how chronic pain can occur and how pain can be felt long after an injury.

This is how neuroplasticity — changes in how your brain responds to pain — can ultimately cause central sensitization. Although the pain may be gone, the nerves that told your brain about it in the first place are still "turned on" — in other words, these nerves are still telling your brain about pain long after it's actually gone. In attempting to cope and help by sending these messages to your brain, your nervous system actually creates more pain, fatigue and other symptoms.

'Pain prone' phenotype

Some people with central sensitization have what's called a "pain prone" phenotype. This means that they're more likely to experience chronic pain after a trauma, injury or stressful period.

Genetics

In some cases, people with central sensitization have a family history of chronic pain. This shows that a genetic influence may play a role in this disorder.

It's not always easy to pinpoint a cause of central sensitization, but in the end, it's not necessarily critical to understand the cause before taking steps to treat the disorder. The important point to keep in mind about the potential causes of central sensitization is that a mix of factors seem to be involved. Nerves may become re-wired for a number of reasons, including adverse experiences during childhood, a mood disorder or having higher levels of stress hormones coursing through your veins.

In the end, no matter the cause, the important point to remember about central sensitization is that it's not something imaginary. Central sensitization is a physical sensory process that works itself into higher levels of stimulus and distress over time. It may not be something that can be physically seen or detected, but these sensations are real and can be treated.

Central sensitization: An endless loop

As you've learned already, central sensitization causes your nerves to keep sending signals to your brain, telling it over and over again about pain in your body, even long after it's gone.

In an effort to protect you, your brain causes your body to react to sensations that pain can cause. You read about these symptoms earlier in this section (starting on page 183). The more your brain hears about these symptoms, the worse the symptoms become.

This is the endless loop of central sensitization. Your brain gets messages about pain that's no longer there, your brain tells your body how to cope with it, and this line of communication gets stronger and stronger over time, worsening the symptoms of central sensitization. Here are four reasons why this happens.

1. Chemical confusion

Many people with central sensitization are given different medications to help treat their many symptoms. Doctors may prescribe pain medications and sleep aids, as well as nerve medications, antidepressants and digestive medications.

As more medications are prescribed to treat the many different specific symptoms that central sensitization can cause, the brain can get confused chemically. In the end, this can make central sensitization worse.

2. Pain behaviors

If you hurt, you may stop doing certain things. Or, on days when you don't hurt as much, you may do too much and hurt more later on. On the other hand, resting too much can lead to physical deconditioning and weakness.

Doing too little or doing too much in response to how much pain you feel are examples of pain behaviors — things that you do, say or think that remind you of your pain. These behaviors can all make central sensitization worse.

3. Emotional distress

Emotions are a response to central sensitization. The more emotional distress the brain experiences, the more sensory or physical distress it will experience, as well. In short, emotional distress keeps central sensitization going.

It's normal to experience emotional distress when you have symptoms you can't understand or manage, especially when they're interfering with your life. That's why symptoms of depression, anxiety and stress are so common in central sensitization. This is also why it's critical to

manage these symptoms — to help tone down these signals to your brain.

4. Loss of physical functioning

Symptoms of central sensitization can make it difficult for people to be able to do things physically — or to feel like they don't want to move at all, in some cases. This makes physical therapy just as important as treating the emotional and chemical issues caused by central sensitization.

Treatment

Medically, it's not possible to shut off central sensitization as you do a light switch. However, you can take steps toward turning down the signals that keep central sensitization going.

Retrain your brain

Earlier in this book (see page 42), you learned that neuroplasticity means you can create new connections in your brain. Practicing a new language or learning how to play a musical instrument are two examples of how you can train your brain. With time, the more you practice a musical instrument, for example, the more you strengthen the connections in your brain that make it possible for you to play that musical instrument. The same goes for any other skill that you learn about and practice so that you can master it.

In central sensitization, as you learned earlier in this section, the same type of change happens in your brain, although not in a good way. As you've learned in this section, for any number of reasons, changes in the nervous system can cause you to feel overly sensitive to pain, making it feel as though pain is still there even if your physical healing is complete. Your brain is trying to protect you from the pain it thinks is present, even though it's not physically there.

Although central sensitization can be considered as a negative example of neuroplasticity, it's important to note that your brain's ability to rewire itself can help treat central sensitization, too. Neuroplasticity can turn down overactive pain signals and all of the symptoms they cause. By cutting off the influences of central sensitization, you can turn down the messages to your brain so that it understands that the body is not under attack and in need of protection.

At Mayo Clinic's interdisciplinary pain rehabilitation centers, pain experts help patients cope with and manage the symptoms of central sensitization with the same techniques that are used to help manage chronic pain. These techniques help settle down the nervous system, which is key to turning down the signals that are causing the symptoms. You'll recognize some of these techniques as integrative therapies that you've already learned about in this book.

Learn more about Mayo Clinic's pain rehabilitation programs and the integrative therapies they use on page 193.

Sleep

More and more research links a good night's sleep to changes in the structure and function of the brain — in other words, neuroplasticity. Sleep supports the learning process that takes place when you're training your brain to do something new. This makes sleep critical to treating symptoms of central sensitization.

Although a good night's sleep will not magically cure central sensitization, it can reduce your experience of pain. In addition, the neuroplastic changes that occur during sleep can be helpful. This is because as you learn to manage your symptoms through the other techniques discussed here, sleep supports the changes you're making to your brain and help them "stick." Most adults need 7 to 8 hours of sleep each night.

Relaxation

Everyone experiences stress, but the challenges of a chronic condition, such as central sensitization, can add more stress.

Stress can worsen symptoms, causing you to tense your muscles, grit your teeth or stiffen your shoulders. This can lead to more pain, and more limits on your ability to handle everyday tasks. Frustration, anger, depression and more tension

Relaxation exercises to treat pain

As you've already learned in this book, relaxation is important to good health. When you are relaxed, your muscles are loose, your heart rate is normal, and your breathing is slow and deep.

In terms of chronic pain, relaxation exercises can be especially helpful, because they release chemicals that reduce pain and produce a sense of well-being.

Relaxation exercises won't magically cure any chronic condition, but learning skills that relax the body and mind is one step you can take to help loosen tense muscles, prevent muscle spasms, and relieve stress that can make pain and other symptoms worse.

And there's one more bonus to relaxation exercises: You don't need any special equipment to do them, and you can do them anytime, anywhere. Learn more about the benefits of relaxation starting on page 43.

Mayo Clinic's interdisciplinary pain rehabilitation programs include structured relaxation, performed on a regular basis each day. Relaxation exercises often introduced in these pain rehabilitation programs include:

- Deep breathing (see page 46)
- Biofeedback (see page 66)
- Progressive muscle relaxation (see page 44)
- Guided visualization (see page 64)
- Meditation (see page 56)
- Yoga (see page 29)
- Tai chi (see page 29)

Remember: Relaxation is a skill that requires time and practice. If you don't see results from practicing a relaxation technique, keep trying. This may mean trying different techniques until you find the right one for you.

Above all, remember that the point of relaxation exercises is to increase your sense of peace and calmness. Learning to use these techniques when you notice signs and symptoms of stress can help you keep stress from spiraling out of control.

often result. With time and practice, relaxation exercises can help you release the tension in your body and lessen the effects of stress, helping to improve your health and your quality of life.

Relaxation is more than having peace of mind, resting or enjoying a hobby. It means eliminating tension from your body and your mind and involves taking a break from your daily tasks to purposefully eliminate tension from your body and mind.

Practicing relaxation techniques, such as relaxed breathing and progressive muscle relaxation, can help relieve stress that can make chronic pain worse. Learn more about the benefits of relaxation exercises, as well as relaxation exercises you can try, starting on page 43.

Exercise

It's a common myth that exercise makes pain worse. In reality, *avoiding* activity can cause you to become deconditioned, which can increase your pain. Exercise can relieve pain, as well as ease depression and anxiety. Activity can also improve your mood and your overall health. Regular exercise increases your flexibility, strength and endurance. It improves your overall fitness. An exercise program can help you live a more active, enjoyable life with less pain.

At Mayo Clinic's interdisciplinary pain rehabilitation programs, experts recommend including three types of exercise in a physical activity plan:
1. Range-of-motion exercises, gentle stretches or other warm-up activities
2. Aerobic exercise
3. Muscle strengthening, stretching and flexibility exercises

Moderation

The longer you've been in pain, the more deconditioned you likely are. And if you're experiencing central sensitization, your pain nerves are more active than normal.

This combination means that you may get fatigued and sore easily. It also means that at first, it may be difficult to overcome your physical deconditioning.

In these cases, people sometimes have a tendency to overdo physical activity, and this can make everything — the pain, fatigue and soreness — worse. A vicious cycle of trying too hard and then not trying at all because of pain ensues. This is where moderation can help.

With moderation, you decide how much, how long, and how quickly you do things so that you avoid doing too much or doing too little during your day. Moderating your activities can help you accomplish daily tasks without increasing pain and other symptoms.

How you organize and conduct your day can affect how well you manage your pain and other symptoms. When you use moderation, you conserve extra energy when you're feeling good so that you can continue your daily activities on days when you have pain, fatigue or other symptoms.

By using time management skills, you can develop a routine that minimizes your stress, conserves your energy and helps you achieve balance in your life. In essence, you're using your energy wisely so that you have enough during the times when you're feeling good, but still have enough energy to use when you're not feeling as well. That way, you can continue living your life despite the symptoms you're experiencing on any given day.

Pacing

As you've learned, central sensitization causes the nervous system to become overstimulated. Doing too much, too soon, can make this worse. For that reason — especially if you haven't been physically active on a regular basis — it's important to start slowly and increase slowly, to set moderate goals, and not attempt to push past them. Pacing goes hand in hand with moderation.

What about medication?

As with other chronic conditions, conventional medical treatment is an option for central sensitization. However, although there are medication options for central sensitization, this treatment option doesn't work for everyone. And in some

Steps to success with relaxation exercises

Stress management and relaxation skills can help give you mental, emotional and physical energy to cope with chronic symptoms. Use these steps from Mayo Clinic experts to bring peace and a sense of calm into your life through relaxation exercises.

Set a routine
- Set aside time to practice relaxation at least once or twice a day.
- Pair relaxation with a regular activity to help you remember to practice it. For example, you may decide to take six relaxed breaths every time you sit down to eat.
- Practice relaxation exercises at various times throughout the day. In this way, the practice becomes natural and you can use it readily when you feel stressed.

Get comfortable
- When practicing relaxation exercises, use a comfortable chair, sofa, mat or bed, in a quiet, dimly lit location.
- Loosen tight clothing and remove shoes, belt, glasses or contact lenses, if it will help you feel more comfortable.

Focus
- Practice in a quiet, calm environment in which you won't be disrupted or distracted.
- Close your eyes to reduce distractions and improve concentration. Or, if you prefer, keep your eyes open and focus on one spot.
- Move your body as little as possible, changing position only for comfort.

Relax
- Begin and end relaxation practices with relaxed breathing techniques.
- If it's helpful when you're first learning, use relaxation instructions on a CD to guide you. Gradually over time, learn to relax without these instructions so you can practice your relaxation techniques anywhere.
- Do not try to force or resist relaxation. Let it happen naturally and spread throughout your body. You may notice sensations of tingling, floating, warmth and heaviness.

Be patient
- Give yourself time to learn relaxation skills. Practice will help these techniques eventually become automatic.
- Try not to become upset if you have trouble concentrating. It's normal for your mind to wander. If your mind wanders, simply bring it back to the focus of your relaxation exercise.
- Don't worry about how well you are practicing.

Incorporate relaxation into daily life
- Over time, move relaxation practices from planned, quiet settings to "real life."
- The goal is to calm yourself when necessary.
- Use relaxation exercises any time you start to feel stressed or anxious.

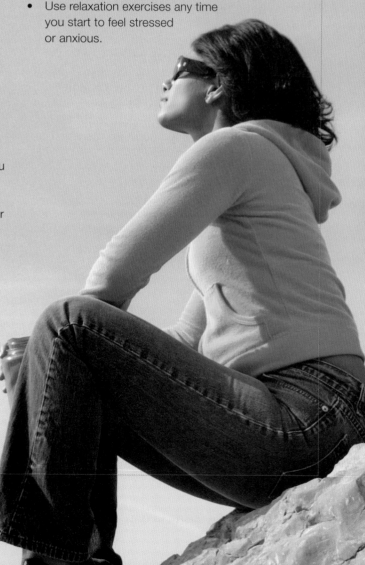

cases, medication can actually make symptoms worse. This is why interdisciplinary pain rehabilitation centers like those at Mayo Clinic focus on the other methods of treatment that you just read about: sleep, exercise, relaxation, moderation and pacing.

With that said, here's what researchers and medical professionals know about medications that have been used to help treat symptoms of central sensitization.

Opioid medications

Opioid medications, which were once used to help treat chronic pain, are no longer recommended for use in treating chronic pain conditions. Even if they were still recommended, they can actually lead to further dysregulation of the same areas that are affected by central sensitization, worsening symptoms.

Fibromyalgia medications

The three FDA-approved medications for the treatment of fibromyalgia may be useful for other forms of central sensitization.

Pregabalin (Lyrica). This anti-convulsant limits the release of pain-communicating chemicals by nerve cells in the brain and spinal cord.

Duloxetine (Cymbalta). This antidepressant is prescribed at a lower dose than what is prescribed for depression.

Milnacipran (Savella). This antidepressant appears to have an additional effect on fatigue, separate from its pain-relieving benefits.

Listen now:

Hear from Brent A. Bauer, M.D., on integrative therapies being used to help treat chronic pain: http://newsnetwork.mayoclinic.org/files/2016/11/Mayo-Clinic-Radio-11-12-16-PODCAST.mp3

Moderation: How to do it

Break up lengthy tasks. Lengthy activities can steal your energy and increase your pain and other symptoms. Instead of spending an entire day doing yardwork, for example, spend one or two hours a day on your outdoor chores over three to four days.

Alternate activities. Instead of filling your day with activities that require the same amount of effort, mix them up. For example, after you've vacuumed one room, sit down and fold laundry or pay bills. Or, after mowing the lawn, sit down and read or watch a movie.

Prioritize tasks. Plan your most important tasks for the times of day when you have the most energy and feel your best.

Take breaks. How often you should take a break depends on the activity. You may find you can do some activities for 30 to 60 minutes before you need a break. More strenuous tasks, such as mowing the lawn, may require a break every 10 to 20 minutes. Be sure to take a break before you become fatigued.

Work at a moderate pace. Working at a fast pace, compared to a moderate pace, requires twice as much energy. Take your time and work at a comfortable speed.

You'll know that your pace is right when you feel as though you're exerting yourself, but not to the point of overdoing it. It may take longer to accomplish a task, but in the end you'll feel better.

Change the frequency of tasks. Some tasks may be less tiring if you break them up and do portions of tasks more often. For example, try doing small loads of laundry three times a week instead of spending several hours doing laundry on one day.

Delegate. If an activity is too difficult or physically demanding, ask for help or assign it to someone else. It isn't always easy to ask for help, but this is one way to ensure that you use your energy wisely.

Interdisciplinary pain rehabilitation programs at Mayo Clinic

Combining conventional and integrative medicine to treat chronic pain

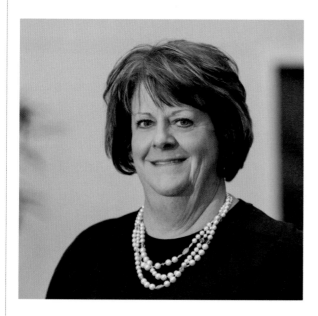

By Barbara K. Bruce, Ph.D., L.P.

Dr. Bruce is the clinical director of Mayo Clinic's Fibromyalgia Treatment Program and its Chronic Abdominal Pain Program, both located at Mayo Clinic in Jacksonville, Florida. Dr. Bruce also directed Mayo Clinic's Comprehensive Pain Rehabilitation Center and created and led Mayo Clinic's Pediatric Pain Rehabilitation Center, both in Rochester, Minnesota.

In 2011, more than 131 million prescriptions were written for hydrocodone, making it the most widely prescribed drug in the United States. Hydrocodone and oxycodone, both examples of opioid pain medications, have fueled an epidemic of addiction and fatal overdoses that outpace those from heroin and cocaine combined.

Taken long term, opioid pain medications are not only dangerous — they also simply aren't effective when it comes to treating chronic pain. Over time, more medication is needed to achieve the same effect, leading to the risk of dependence, addiction, overdose and a reduced quality of life.

These issues have led the Centers for Disease Control and Prevention to no longer recommend opioid medications for treating chronic pain. They also signal a need for a new approach to pain management, making interdisciplinary pain programs such as Mayo Clinic's — the first one of which opened in 1974 — more important than ever. These programs combine conventional medicine with integrative techniques to help people reduce their pain and manage pain more effectively.

Instead of placing an emphasis on a specific area of pain or a group of symptoms, the basis of interdisciplinary pain programs is self-management. Self-management means that you're focusing your body and mind on wellness — and that's where integrative techniques come in. The approach to pain management taught in Mayo Clinic's pain rehabilitation programs combines traditional medical approaches with integrative techniques. In terms of conventional medicine, these programs address:
- The role of medication and other treatments
- Physical and occupational therapy

Integrative therapies taught in Mayo Clinic's pain rehabilitation programs include:
- Techniques for managing stress
- Relaxation exercises
- Practicing positive thinking
- Biofeedback
- Yoga

These topics provide just a sampling of what's covered at the pain rehabilitation programs offered at Mayo Clinic, but they illustrate the importance of ways that conventional medicine and integrative therapies can be used together to help promote health and wellness and improve quality of life.

And this combination seems to be working: Of those who have completed Mayo Clinic's three-week comprehensive pain rehabilitation program, 84 percent say that they're better able to manage their pain, even without medication.

Is integrative medicine right for you?

As you've learned throughout this book, integrative medicine encompasses a diverse group of products, practices and therapies — all intended to be used alongside conventional medicine for treating and preventing illness. As nontraditional approaches to health gain greater acceptance as potential forms of healing, an increasing number are undergoing scientific study. Some are incorporated into mainstream medicine, while others fall out of favor because they're shown to be ineffective or unsafe.

For many integrative practices, however, the jury is still out. Either study results have been inconclusive or not enough research has been conducted to fully determine the therapy's effectiveness and safety.

Integrative medicine — just like any medical treatment — is not without its risks. For the most part, the risks are dependent on the specific therapy. That's why each therapy discussed in this book needs to be considered on its own. You can't assume that because one type of treatment is safe and effective, similar products and practices are as well.

That's why it's important to do your homework. If you're considering a specific therapy, research its safety, be aware of potential side effects, and take steps to minimize risks. And remember, just because a product may be referred to as "natural," that doesn't necessarily guarantee that it's safe. It may contain certain chemicals that don't mix with other medications you're taking. Or it could harbor unknown ingredients. Think of tobacco, strychnine and poison ivy. They're all natural — but they aren't safe!

In this section, you'll learn how to find good information about the therapies you're interested in so that you can evaluate them. You'll also learn how to talk with your health care team about specific products and practices, and how to find a qualified provider if you decide that an integrative approach is right for you.

Finding good research

When it comes to your health, you want to make sure you're basing your decisions on trusted and credible information. Many websites, mobile apps and print publications provide health information, but not all of them are trustworthy. So where do you find good research?

Start your search for information with government agencies, such as the National Institutes of Health (*http://www.ncbi.nlm.nih.gov/pubmed/*), and well-respected hospitals and universities. Evidence-based studies that have been published in medical journals are also credible sources of health information.

What makes a good study?

As you've read through this book, you likely noticed products that haven't been "well-studied," or therapies that need "more-rigorous scientific study." So what makes a good study?

In general, the larger the study, the better. When a study involves several hundred people or more — especially if it lasts over several months or years — it gains more credibility. You've likely also noticed places throughout this book that have highlighted research from "a small study," or research that lasted for a shorter amount of time. In these cases, it's noted that the integrative therapy being discussed needs more research — this, in part, is why.

How the study was performed also is key. Prospective double-blind studies that have been carefully controlled, randomized and published in peer-reviewed journals are the gold standard. What does that mean? Here's some information to help you out.

- **Clinical studies.** Clinical studies are those that involve human beings — not animals. They're usually preceded by studies conducted in animals that demonstrate safety and effectiveness. There are two major types of clinical studies. In an **observational study**, participants are simply observed and no treatment is given. In an **interventional study**, a treatment is given and monitored to learn if it works and

if it's safe. Clinical studies that are rigorously controlled are designed to lead to a significant amount of detailed data that shows how safe — and how helpful — a treatment may be.

- **Randomized controlled trials.** In this type of study, the participants are usually divided randomly into two groups. One group receives the treatment being studied, while the other group receives a placebo treatment. Randomly assigning participants to one of two groups is done to ensure that participants with certain characteristics don't all end up in the same group. Randomly assigning participants into one of two groups is also a way to help balance the unique characteristics of the participants. The first group receives the treatment being studied. The second group is the control group. People in the control group may receive standard treatment, no treatment or an inactive substance called a placebo (see "The placebo effect" on the next page). A randomized trial is one in which participants are assigned to the individual groups on a random basis to help ensure all of the groups will be similar.
- **Double-blind studies.** Blinding a study is a lot like it sounds. In double-blind studies, neither the researchers nor the participants know who is receiving the active treatment or the placebo. This type of study is also known as **double-blind masking**.
- **Prospective studies.** Prospective studies are forward-looking. With these studies, researchers establish criteria for study participants to follow and then measure or describe the results. Information from these studies is usually more reliable than that of retrospective studies.
- **Retrospective studies.** Opposite prospective studies, they involve looking at past data, which leaves room for error in interpretation.
- **Peer-reviewed journals.** These journals publish only articles that have been reviewed by an independent panel of medical experts. The review is usually anonymous, and the reviewers usually aren't paid. Learn if a journal is peer-reviewed by visiting its home

page. There, look for "peer-reviewed" and "acceptance rate." A journal that is peer-reviewed and has an acceptance rate below 20 percent offers the best quality information.

When you're evaluating a scientific study, look for clinical studies that involve human beings, not animals. Mice and men have many genes in common, but a man is still not a mouse. Also check to see how the study was conducted and how many participants were involved.

Finally, ask yourself if the research applies to you. For example, Mayo Clinic has conducted two studies to see if ginseng can lessen fatigue in people who have had cancer. For these studies, the ginseng was obtained from a specific grower in Wisconsin to oversee that harvesting and processing were uniform for all of the ginseng samples. This helped ensure that each capsule contained the same amount of the active ingredients. In this case, studies showed that ginseng helped those in the study group feel less fatigued. But that doesn't necessarily mean it will have the same effect for you. If you're not buying the same type of ginseng and you're not a cancer survivor, you may not see the same results.

When looking at research, seek out not only good-quality studies, but also studies that you can relate to based on your goals for taking a supplement in the first place.

The three D's

When looking for information on integrative medicine or a particular product or therapy, chances are you can find plenty of information — likely more than you need — on the internet. The internet offers a virtually limitless supply of information on all sorts of integrative treatments. But it's also one of the greatest sources of misinformation. As you're doing your homework, weed out the good information from the bad. To do that, use the three D's:

Dates. Check the creation or update date for each article. If you don't see a date, don't assume the article is recent. Older material may be outdated and may not include recent findings.

Documentation. Who operates the site? Are qualified health professionals creating and

The placebo effect

A placebo is a substance or a therapy that appears to be a real medical treatment, but isn't. A placebo could be a pill, a shot or some other type of false treatment. Often, a placebo is a sugar solution without any active ingredients disguised to look like what it's trying to mimic.

What researchers have discovered is that people who think they're getting a real medicine when it's really just a placebo sometimes get better. This remarkable and quite real benefit is called the "placebo effect," and it's a good example of how our minds and beliefs can affect our bodies. When you expect your physical symptoms to improve, they often do — even though you may not be doing or taking anything different.

Improvement due to the placebo effect is improvement, and that's always welcome. But it's important to remember that for many health conditions, there are often treatments that work better than placebo treatments. That's why it's important to test all potential treatments to find out what works best for you.

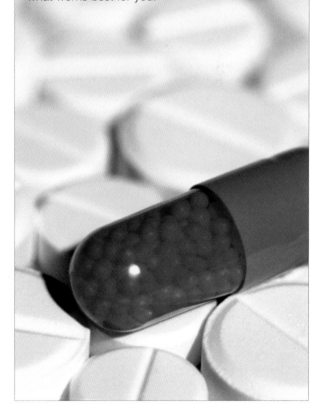

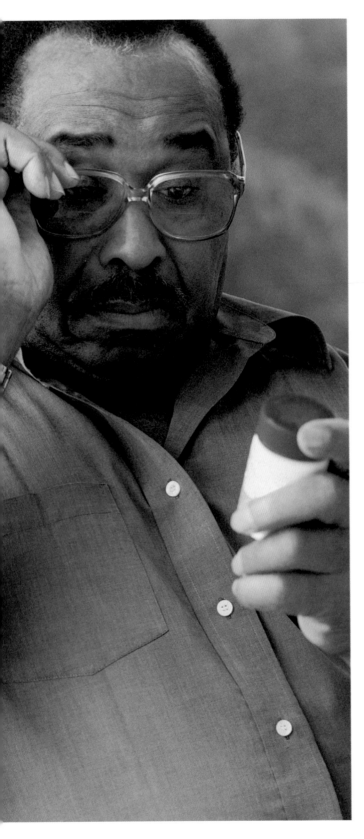

reviewing the information? Are references listed? Is advertising clearly identified? Look for the logo from the Health on the Net (HON) Foundation (*www.healthonnet.org*), which means that the site follows HON's principles for reliability and credibility of information.

Double-check. Visit several health websites and compare the information they offer. If you can't find supporting evidence to back up the claims of an integrative medicine product, be skeptical. And before you follow any advice you read on the internet, check with your health care team for guidance.

Bottom line: If what you read sounds too good to be true, it probably is. Make an effort to seek out additional information from a reliable, authoritative source, and talk with your doctor or another trusted health care professional.

Sound too good to be true? Maybe it is

The Food and Drug Administration (FDA) recommends that you watch for the following claims or practices. These can be warning signs of potentially fraudulent dietary supplements or other so-called "natural" treatments:

- The advertisements and claims seem exaggerated or unrealistic. They may include words such as "breakthrough," "magical" or "new discovery." If the product were in fact a cure, your doctor would recommend it. Also be leery of claims that the product is "totally safe."
- The manufacturer claims that the product can treat a wide range of symptoms — is a "cure-all" — or can cure or prevent a number of diseases. No single product can do this.
- The product is supposedly backed by scientific studies, but references aren't provided. Be skeptical of information that comes from personal testimonials.
- The product claims to be an alternative to an FDA-approved drug or to have effects similar to prescription drugs.
- The product is marketed primarily through mass emails or is marketed primarily in a foreign language.

What you need to know about dietary supplements

If you've walked through a health food store or even down the nutrition aisle of your local grocery store or pharmacy, you know all too well that the number of herbal remedies and other dietary supplements is overwhelming.

A 2015 consumer safety survey conducted by the Council for Responsible Nutrition found that more than two-thirds of Americans take dietary supplements, including vitamins and minerals. Dietary supplements are by far the most common form of complementary medicine, accounting for nearly one-fifth of all integrative therapy in the United States.

That same 2015 consumer safety survey also found that the vast majority of people who take supplements consider them to be safe and effective. What's important to know is that supplements are not the same as medications. The companies that manufacture supplements are not subject to the same regulations as those that manufacture drugs.

Limited regulation

In 1994, the U.S. Congress passed the Dietary Supplement Health and Education Act (DSHEA). This legislation was originally proposed by the Food and Drug Administration (FDA) to enhance oversight of supplement manufacturers in response to serious adverse effects traced back to specific herbs and supplements. But the industry pushed back, and eventually, Congress passed the DSHEA. The DSHEA created the category of "dietary supplements," and in the end, resulted in a lot less oversight power than what was originally proposed.

There are two critical parts of the dietary supplements act that deserve special attention.
• Manufacturers do not have to prove efficacy. That means they aren't required to conduct formal research to prove that their product does what they claim.
• Manufacturers don't have to prove the safety of their products. They're expected to have

some historical usage data to support its safety, but again, there's no requirement for specific testing to ensure a product is safe.

With these exemptions in place, the supplement market blossomed. At the same time, there was growing dissatisfaction with the current state of medicine in the United States. Patients and consumers wanted to be more engaged in their care, and the boom in supplement sales was partly due to that search for greater health care autonomy.

This isn't meant to suggest that the FDA isn't regulating the supplements market. The agency does a lot to make sure the products you buy are safe and of high quality. However, the rules that Congress passed limit the FDA in many ways. That's why consumers need to choose wisely when adding dietary supplements to their daily regimens.

Ensuring the quality of herbs and supplements sold in the U.S. is a challenge. In numerous cases, people have been harmed by products that included the wrong herb or that contained actual prescription drugs. Many herbal remedies produced in China, for example, have been found to contain toxic amounts of heavy metals, such as arsenic, lead and mercury.

Today, thanks to rules implemented in 2010 called Good Manufacturing Practices (GMPs), all supplements sold in the U.S. are now mandated to contain exactly what's stated on the label. However, there are still some bad actors out there, mostly fly-by-night internet setups. That's why despite GMPs, it's important that you know what to look for to ensure that you're purchasing good-quality products.

Safe use

How can you make sure you're getting good-quality products and you're taking them correctly? Follow these safety guidelines:
• **Tell your doctor what you're taking.** Some

supplements may interfere with the effectiveness of prescription medications you're taking or have other harmful effects. It's always a good idea to keep your doctor informed of everything you take.

- **Read the label and look for a seal of approval.** An example is the U.S. Pharmacopeia's "USP Dietary Supplement Verified" mark. It indicates that a product meets certain standards of quality. Other groups that certify supplements include ConsumerLab.com and NSF International. Although each group takes a slightly different approach, the goal of each is to certify that the product meets a certain standard.
- **Choose a name you know.** Look for a large, recognizable manufacturer. While this isn't a guarantee that the product contains exactly what it says it does, chances are better that a well-known company with a good reputation will make the effort to produce a quality product.
- **Follow the directions.** Herbal products have active ingredients that can affect how your body functions. Don't exceed the recommended dosages.
- **Be cautious about products manufactured or purchased outside the United States.** Some European herbs are well-regulated and standardized. But toxic ingredients (including lead and mercury) and prescription drugs (such as prednisone) have been found in herbal supplements manufactured elsewhere, particularly China, India and Mexico.
- **Avoid supplements if you're pregnant or breast-feeding.** Only take supplements if your doctor says it's OK. They could harm the baby.
- **Stay away from potentially dangerous herbs.** Know which herbs are dangerous and can be fatal. Some examples include chaparral, ephedra (ma-huang) and kava. Although some of these supplements are "banned," they're still available on the internet.

When medicines and supplements don't mix

What happens when you mix herbs with prescription or nonprescription medications? The truth is, we often don't know. Researchers are studying this question and hope to have a better understanding of these interactions in the future. For the time being, the best advice is to think twice before mixing any herb with a prescription or nonprescription drug.

Supplements of concern

Certain supplements have been recognized as having a high risk of interactions with certain medications. You don't want to mix medications with these particular herbs without your doctor's approval because of potential risks. Some supplements of concern include:

- Black cohosh
- Dong quai
- Evening primrose oil
- Garlic
- Ginkgo
- Ginseng
- Hawthorn
- Kava
- St. John's wort
- Yohimbe

Medications of concern

Some medications have what's called a *narrow therapeutic window*. If their level is too low or too high, problems can occur. An example is the anticoagulant medication warfarin (Coumadin). If the medication level is too low, dangerous blood clotting can occur. If the level is too high, dangerous bleeding can occur.

If you're taking warfarin, it's important that other drugs you take — including vitamins and supplements — not interfere with the therapeutic window of the drug.

Other medications with narrow therapeutic windows include those that control heart arrhythmias, prevent organ rejection and control seizures.

Talking with your health care team

After you've done your homework and you feel like you have the information you need to talk with your health care team about the integrative therapy you'd like to try, it's time to take the next step. Together with your health care team, discuss the information you've found, talk about your health history, and decide if the therapy makes sense and is safe for you.

This may sound simpler than if feels, however. You may be unsure about talking with your doctor about nontraditional therapies for a variety of reasons. Perhaps you're worried that he or she will criticize you or think that you've lost all good sense. If the therapy isn't dangerous, this shouldn't be the case. Most doctors are well aware that unconventional products and practices are highly popular, and they want to help their patients use these therapies safely. Other changes have taken place in the past several years that may help make your conversation a little easier, too.

For example, in the last 20 years, more scientific studies on nontraditional treatments have been — and continue to be — conducted. This research gives doctors more confidence in recommending certain therapies. Today, if a doctor wants to know more about a certain therapy or if a patient has questions, he or she often can look at data in a peer-reviewed study.

Another change in the health care system is the doctor-patient relationship. It's become more of a partnership. Because patients today are more educated and ask more questions than they used to, doctors have had to learn different ways of thinking and interacting with their patients — including treatments that may not always follow conventional practices.

A third difference in medicine today is the shift in focus from preventive medicine toward wellness. This is where integrative practices can play a huge role. Conventional medicine can help treat health issues that already exist, but it isn't always suited to preventing future problems. Managing stress, eating a healthy diet and getting plenty of exercise are all ways to help prevent a heart attack from happening in the first place, for example. When combined with conventional medicine, integrative practices can help individuals reduce stress, eat well and improve overall health. That means they can also potentially help prevent problems before they have a chance to start.

For these reasons, health care professionals are gradually becoming more open to the idea of integrative medicine. For instance, medical students today are largely following natural diets and eating organic foods more often, and their parents may be practicing tai chi. These days, it's not uncommon to see medical students participating in yoga sessions before class or meditating together.

Act sooner, rather than later

Try not to put off your discussion about integrative therapies. It's best to talk with your health care team *before* you begin a new therapy instead of after you get started. Why? Team members can help you think through a number of issues. Your doctor or other members of your team can:

- Identify if a treatment has any potentially dangerous side effects
- Let you know if a product may interact with a medication you currently use
- Help you determine the correct dosage
- Confirm that the therapy seems appropriate for you and your needs
- Put you in touch with someone who performs the therapy you're interested in, or who can teach you how to do it

During the conversation with your doctor, be honest. Answer his or her questions truthfully so that he or she can accurately monitor your health, assess any potential health risks and get you off to a good start.

Finding a qualified practitioner

When seeking out an integrative health practitioner, be as careful and thorough as you were when you were searching for your primary care physician. When you're searching for a provider, the

National Center for Complementary and Integrative Health recommends taking these steps:

- **To locate practitioners in your area, first check with your doctor or other health care provider.** A nearby hospital or medical school, professional organizations, state regulatory agencies or licensing boards, or even your health insurance provider also may be helpful.
- **Find out as much as you can about the person's education, training, licensing and certifications.** Credentials required for integrative health practitioners vary from state to state and from discipline to discipline.

Once you've found a possible practitioner, ask yourself these questions to determine if the individual is right for you:

- **Is he or she willing to work together with your conventional health care providers?** For safe, coordinated care, all of the professionals involved in your care should communicate and cooperate.

- **Does his or her training and experience align with my condition and concerns?** Select a practitioner who understands how to care for your specific needs, even if general well-being is your goal.
- **Are his or her services covered by my health insurance?** Contact your health insurance provider and ask. Insurance plans differ greatly in what integrative health approaches they cover, and even if they cover a particular approach, restrictions may apply.

After your first visit, assess the individual and the care you received and decide if this practitioner is right for you and the treatment plan is reasonable. Once you've decided on a complementary provider, make sure to let your health care team know about this person and the treatment that you're receiving. To provide the best care possible, it's important that your primary care team know about all of the health care providers you see.

Understand the unease

When it comes to nontraditional medicine, don't be surprised if your doctor is cautious about endorsing or embracing certain products or practices. Often, this is because the therapy lacks good scientific study. Understandably, the more evidence there is to support a particular product or practice, the more comfortable doctors feel in recommending it.

Also, don't forget that many people have been harmed — in some cases even killed — by products that have been touted as miracle cures or safe alternatives to conventional care.

It's heart-wrenching for any health professional to see, for instance, a young woman with easily treatable breast cancer turn away from conventional medicine because she's been told of the horrors of chemotherapy, only to take an unconventional, unproven treatment and then return to the doctor's office six months later with a more-advanced cancer that now requires more-complicated treatment — or worse yet, is no longer treatable.

Doctors who have seen this type of harm might be more leery of integrative therapies. If your doctor happens to fall into this category, recognize that he or she may have had an unfortunate past experience with a patient that has produced skepticism.

If possible, ask for a referral to a specialist who's knowledgeable in this area or seek out a second opinion from another medical professional.

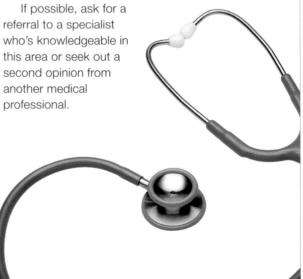

Personal perspectives

Throughout the pages of this book, you have learned about several types of integrative medicine and how they work. Now, we turn to two real-life stories of Mayo Clinic patients who have experienced integrative medicine. Their stories represent different ways integrative medicine can be used to help treat a variety of conditions.

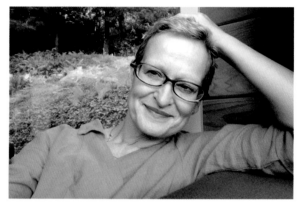

Annemieke van der Werff

When Annemieke van der Werff learned she had breast cancer, she knew she needed a plan to manage her stress. So just before she started treatment, Annemieke stopped at the Mayo Clinic Store in Rochester, Minnesota, and picked up a CD featuring stress reduction exercises. This was ultimately Annemieke's first step toward a meditation practice that she continues to this day.

During chemotherapy, meditation — specifically, mindfulness-based stress reduction — was one way Annemieke felt she could give back to her body while going through treatment. It also helped her focus on enjoying life, whether she was walking through the woods, reading a book or visiting with friends, which always involves great healthy cooking.

With cancer treatment behind her, Annemieke still meditates daily. Depending on the day, she may sit in silent meditation in morning, focusing on her breath and her body. Or, she might meditate while hiking or practice guided meditation with a total body scan.

"I feel very happy and healthy," Annemieke says. "Life is good."

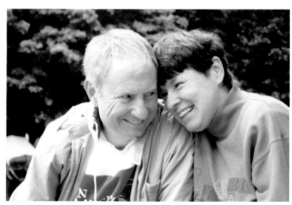

Bill Hunt and Mary Friedel-Hunt

Very suddenly one day, Bill Hunt became anxious and began trembling uncontrollably. "His symptoms came on so quickly, I was sure he had a serious neurological disorder," says Bill's wife, Mary Friedel-Hunt. But extensive testing came back negative. Bill and Mary were told that Bill's loss of some cognitive abilities was a result of amyloid angiopathy and mild brain atrophy. This, combined with emotional stress, led to his shaking and anxiety. In their search to treat Bill's shaking, the Hunts came to the Mayo Clinic Integrative Medicine and Health Program and met with Amit Sood, M.D., who recommended that Bill try mindfulness meditation.

Bill's prescription was to totally focus on an object for 15 minutes several times a day. After one session, Bill's shaking stopped. He continued using mindfulness several times a day, in combination with other suggestions from Dr. Sood.

Integrative medicine helped Bill find meaning and passion to propel him into useful activities. Although Bill has since died, Mary continues the mindfulness meditation that they practiced together to this day.

Talking points to get you started

Once you feel prepared and ready to talk about integrative medicine with your health care team for your specific situation and the goals you would like to reach, you may want help getting the discussion started. This form may help.

Many health care institutions use a form similar to this for patients who are visiting an integrative medicine department for the first time. When used with a complete medical history, filling out a form like this can help you think through the types of integrative medicine you'd like to discuss, why you would like to try them, and what you are hoping to accomplish in adding integrative medicine therapies to your overall wellness plan.

Make a copy of this worksheet, complete it and take it to your next appointment with your health care team to get your conversation about integrative medicine started.

What are the main topics you would like to address today?
Select up to four topics that are concerning you most.
- ○ Pain
- ○ Fatigue
- ○ Stress
- ○ Anxiety
- ○ Fibromyalgia
- ○ Sleep problems
- ○ Cancer
- ○ Heart disease
- ○ Other(s) _____

Which parts of your life are affected by these issues?
- ○ Work
- ○ Sleep
- ○ Eating
- ○ Relationships
- ○ Energy
- ○ Mood
- ○ Other(s) _____

_____

What are your goals for this visit?

_____

_____

_____

What integrative medicine therapies do you already use or have you tried? (Examples include supplements, meditation, acupuncture, massage.)

_____

_____

General health

On average, how would you describe your overall health?
○ Excellent ○ Very good ○ Good ○ Fair ○ Poor

On average, how would you describe your diet?
○ Excellent ○ Very good ○ Good ○ Fair ○ Poor

On average, what is your usual level of physical activity?
- ○ Almost no activity (mainly sitting)
- ○ Mild activity (walking short periods, not lifting or carrying)
- ○ Moderate activity (walking a lot, not lifting or carrying)
- ○ Heavy activity (usually running, lifting or carrying)

On average, how would you describe your sleep?
○ Excellent ○ Very good ○ Good ○ Fair ○ Poor

How would you rate your energy level?
- ○ Very low
- ○ Low
- ○ Moderate
- ○ High
- ○ Very high

Emotional well-being

How would you rate your stress level?
- ○ Very low
- ○ Low
- ○ Moderate
- ○ High
- ○ Very high

How would you rate your anxiety level?
- ○ Very low
- ○ Low
- ○ Moderate
- ○ High
- ○ Very high

What are the biggest stressors in your life?

_____

_____

_____

_____

What steps do you take to cope with stress?

_____

_____

_____

_____

How often do you practice a relaxation program?
- ○ Not at all
- ○ A few times a month
- ○ A few times a week
- ○ Most days of the week
- ○ Every day

Which relaxation programs do you practice? (Mark all that apply.)
- ○ Prayer
- ○ Meditation
- ○ Yoga
- ○ Guided imagery
- ○ Deep breathing
- ○ Music
- ○ Art
- ○ Reading

Meaning and purpose

What brings you joy and meaning in your life?

_____

_____

_____

On average, how would you describe your spiritual well-being?
○ Excellent ○ Very good ○ Good ○ Fair ○ Poor

On average, how would you describe your relationships?
○ Excellent ○ Very good ○ Good ○ Fair ○ Poor

On average, how would you describe your work-life balance?
○ Excellent ○ Very good ○ Good ○ Fair ○ Poor

Next steps

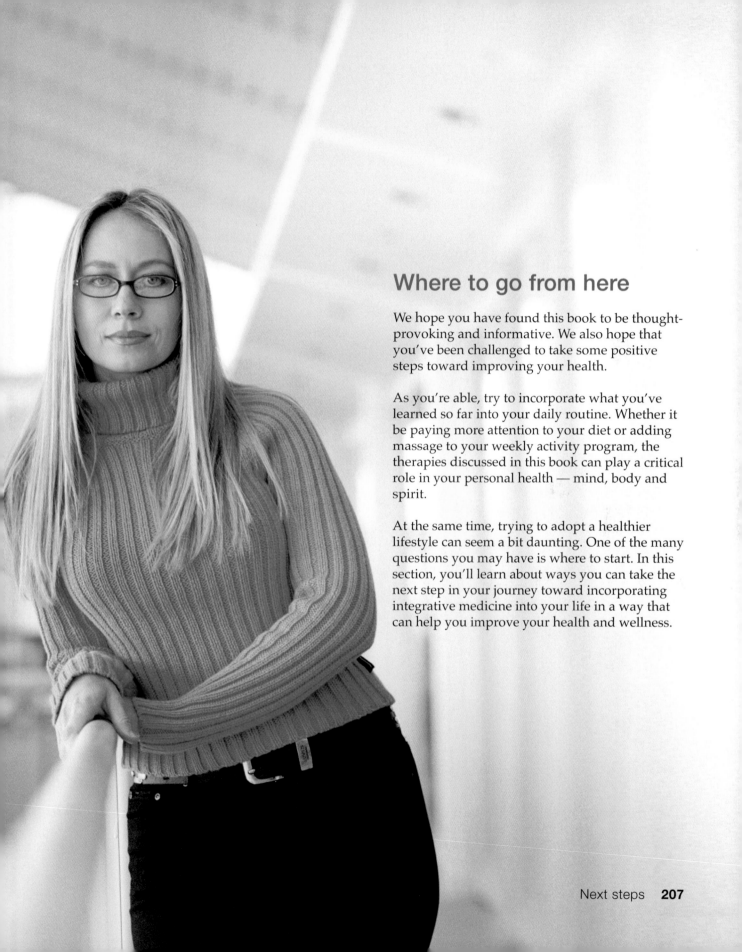

Where to go from here

We hope you have found this book to be thought-provoking and informative. We also hope that you've been challenged to take some positive steps toward improving your health.

As you're able, try to incorporate what you've learned so far into your daily routine. Whether it be paying more attention to your diet or adding massage to your weekly activity program, the therapies discussed in this book can play a critical role in your personal health — mind, body and spirit.

At the same time, trying to adopt a healthier lifestyle can seem a bit daunting. One of the many questions you may have is where to start. In this section, you'll learn about ways you can take the next step in your journey toward incorporating integrative medicine into your life in a way that can help you improve your health and wellness.

5 strategies for moving forward

Are you ready to take an integrative approach to your health? Apply what you've learned in this book with these five steps.

1. Make a commitment

Whether you are a seasoned yoga practitioner or are taking a first step into the realm of wellness, make improving your health a priority.

Often, people find that writing down goals can help them make — and keep — healthy habits. Because life can get hectic and personal wellness may end up at the bottom of your list of priorities, you may find it helpful to mark down your commitment where you can see it every day — to make it an appointment like you do anything else that's important to remember. For example, add 30 minutes of tai chi at 7 a.m. to your calendar a few days a week, or 20 minutes of meditation each night before you go to bed.

2. Start small

Choose one or two therapies from this book that resonate with you — or that target an area of concern. For example, if you have fibromyalgia, adding a weekly massage to your wellness regimen may be a good first step.

Keep in mind that if you start off trying to do too much at one time, you might get overwhelmed and discouraged. Instead, start small. If your goal is to improve your eating habits, a gradual approach may be to try adding one serving of a favorite fruit or vegetable to your current diet three times a week. After a month, aim for a serving of one new fruit or vegetable each week in place of a less-healthy snack. Try different approaches until you find what works best for you.

3. Stick with it

None of the approaches in this book will create significant changes in your health overnight. In some cases, it may take several weeks before you begin to see benefits. Try to give any new therapy at least four to six weeks to pay off.

4. Reassess

Once you've made a change, ask yourself if the change is helping you as much as you'd hoped that it would. If the answer is yes, keep going! If you're not seeing the improvements you'd hoped to see, don't despair. Talk with your doctor or an instructor to see if there are things you can do that might yield better results. If you still don't see benefits, it may be time to try something else. Keep exploring until you find practices that fit you and your needs.

5. Grow

Nurture all aspects of your life — mind, body and spirit. If you started out small, you stuck with it, and you're finding that a certain integrative therapy is helping you, it may be time to expand. Consider selecting another area of your personal wellness that might benefit from greater attention, and follow the same steps — make a commitment, start small, stick with it and then reassess.

At the same time, realize that people are generally drawn to something new. If what you have been doing for a period of time doesn't have the same spark for you that it once did, trying something new may be just what you need to reinvigorate your wellness routine.

Ideally, this book has illustrated why therapies such as massage, meditation and acupuncture are valuable. Now it's up to you to find out what meets your individual needs and fits your personal lifestyle.

One more note: Make your journey into integrative medicine a team effort. Talk with your health care team about what you've learned. From there, work together to make sure any changes you're contemplating won't interfere with the good care you're already receiving.

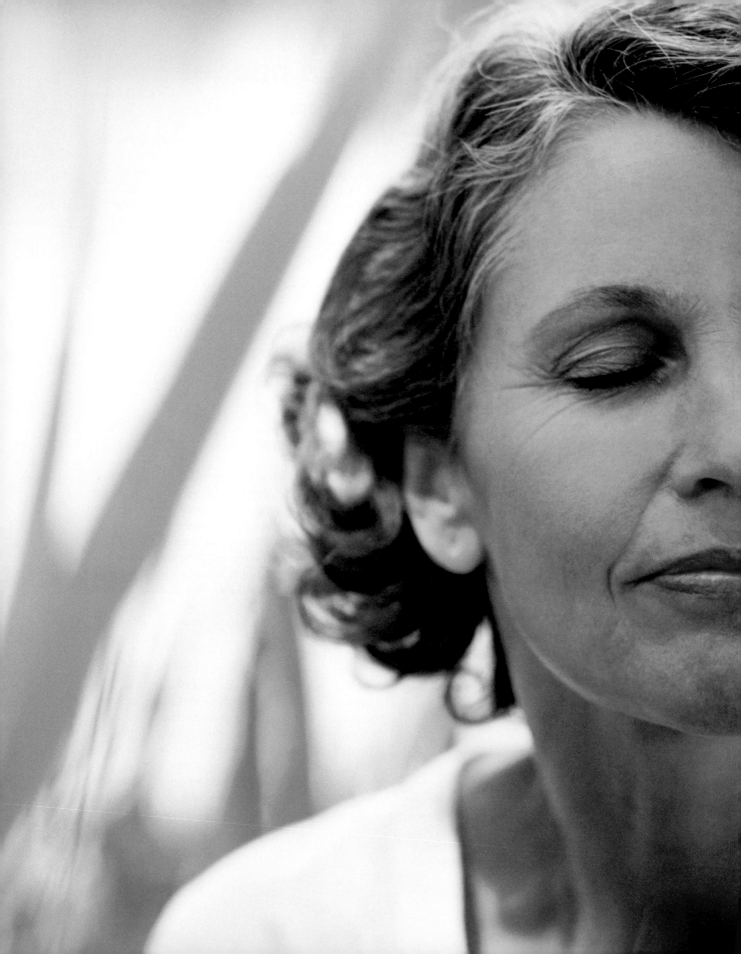

Integrative medicine on a budget

Affordability is a significant issue for many people when it comes to health care, so understandably, you may question if integrative medicine is a type of therapy that can fit into your lifestyle from a cost perspective.

While it's true that some integrative therapies, such as massage and acupuncture, do involve cost, many do not. Here is a list of integrative medicine techniques that cost little or nothing that you can do on your own.

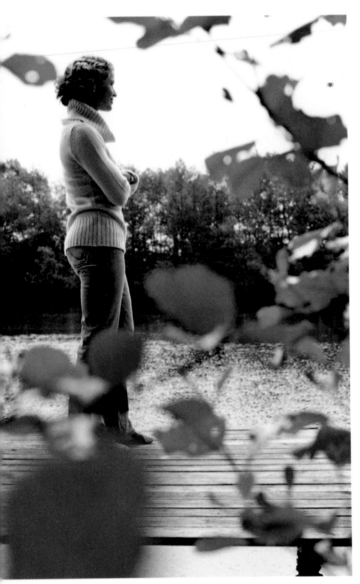

Art therapy

Whether you're drawing, painting, sculpting or producing art in another form, creating art or even interpreting artwork can be therapeutic. With art therapy, you can spend as little or as much money as you'd like to find the medium that works best for you. Learn more about art therapy on page 48.

Deep breathing

Breathing is something you do naturally without giving it much thought. But by breathing through your diaphragm, slowly and deeply, you can experience the stress-relieving benefits of this integrative therapy. Learn more about deep breathing on page 46.

Guided imagery

Your imagination is a powerful thing, and it's already built into your brain and ready for you to use. Guided imagery involves forming mental images of places or situations you find relaxing. For the cost of a CD, you can receive instructions that you can listen to, prompting you to use all of your senses to imagine a scene that brings you a sense of peacefulness. Learn more about guided imagery on page 64.

Meditation

At its core, meditation is a practice of focusing your attention on something that helps you achieve a state of physical relaxation, mental calmness and psychological balance. Maybe your focus is on your breathing, as you inhale and exhale, or on a specific word that you're repeating. Or maybe you meditate by taking a moment of gratitude before you sit down at your desk. Learn more about meditation on page 56.

Pilates

With nothing more than a mat, you can practice Pilates as an integrative technique both for physical activity and stress relief, as well as other health and wellness benefits. If Pilates is new for you, talk to your doctor about it and get guidance from an instructor first. Learn more about Pilates on page 29.

Positive thinking

How you view the world around you and the everyday events in your life can make a significant difference in your overall well-being — and changing your thoughts costs you nothing. Learn about positive thinking and how you can use it to reframe your thoughts on page 75.

Progressive muscle relaxation

Tensing and relaxing each of your muscle groups in sequence can help you find — and release — tension in your body. Learn more about progressive muscle relaxation on page 44.

Qi gong

A Chinese medicine practice that generally combines meditation, relaxation, physical movement and breathing exercises, qi gong is designed to restore and maintain balance. Learn how qi gong represents a type of integrative physical activity that can promote health and wellness on page 29.

Spirituality

No matter how you experience spirituality, finding a way to connect with yourself and others, develop your personal value system, and search for meaning in life are all ways you can improve your wellness and quality of life. Learn more about spirituality on page 72.

Tai chi

Tai chi is a self-paced, mind-body intervention that involves performing a series of postures or movements in a slow, graceful manner while practicing deep breathing. Tai chi requires no special equipment and can be done anywhere — indoors or outside, alone or in a group class.

Although you can rent or buy videos and read books about tai chi, consider seeking guidance from a qualified tai chi instructor to gain the full benefits and learn proper techniques. In addition, it's important to talk to your doctor first before trying tai chi — although it's generally safe, people with certain conditions may need to take extra precautions. Learn how tai chi represents a type of integrative physical activity that can promote health and wellness on page 29.

Yoga

Offering benefits for both physical and mental health, yoga involves performing a series of postures and controlled breathing exercises designed to promote a more flexible body and a calm mind. As you move through poses that require balance and concentration, you're encouraged to focus less on your busy day and more on the moment.

Although you can learn yoga from books and videos, beginners usually find it helpful to learn with an instructor. Speaking of beginners, if you are new to yoga, talk to your doctor first. Yoga is generally safe for most healthy people when it's practiced under the guidance of a trained instructor, but in some situations, yoga may pose risks. Learn how yoga represents a type of integrative physical activity that can promote health and wellness on page 29.

Transforming your health and your future

As you move forward in your wellness journey and consider ways that integrative health practices can play a role in your health, think about the things you can do each day to enhance your well-being. Think of the basics that you learned about at the beginning of this book: nutrition, exercise, stress management and support. What do you do each day to support your wellness in these areas? From eating the right foods and exercising regularly to meditating and even spending time at a spa, every effort you make to improve your overall physical and mental health helps not just you, but also your family and even your community.

Healthy habits have a powerful ripple effect. Look around to see what you can do to integrate the best complementary practices with the best of conventional medicine to achieve a lifetime of health and wellness.

Want to know more?

At the end of this book, you'll find a number of resources where you can obtain more-detailed information from trusted and reliable agencies and organizations. Also visit our website at *www.MayoClinic.org*.

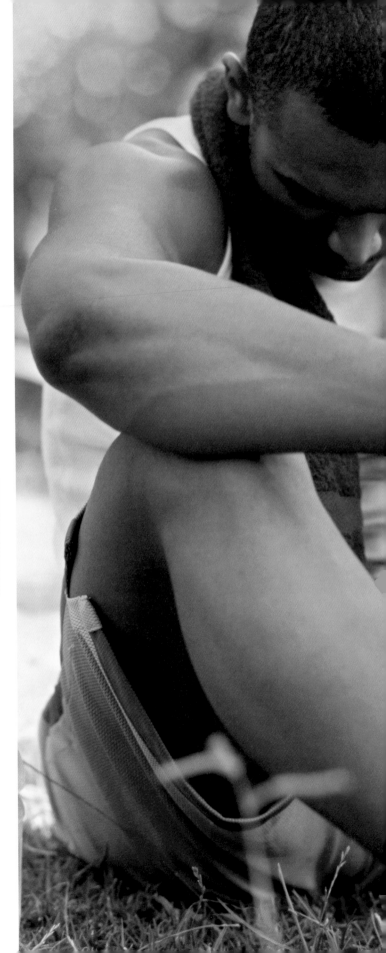

Wellness: Latest developments, what's up next

In this book, you've learned about how integrative medicine can play a role in helping you build a strong wellness foundation that can give you the opportunity to live life to the best of your ability. Years of research have gone into wellness — namely, what wellness truly means and how it can be achieved. Here's a sampling of insights into what medical experts know about what constitutes wellness now — as well as what's on the horizon.

Lessons from the 'Blue Zones'

Research conducted by Dan Buettner, working with National Geographic and a team of scientists and organizations that specialize in aging, found that people in certain areas of the world tend to live longer, healthier, happier lives and experience very few of the diseases that affect others. In these areas of the world, called Blue Zones, people are three times as likely as most Americans to live to be 100 years old, and still enjoy life.

Researchers, anthropologists, demographers and epidemiologists involved in the Blue Zones project found clear and common reasons why these people live longer, healthier, happier lives, and those reasons probably won't surprise you. People in the Blue Zones:

- Stay in motion throughout the day
- Have a sense of purpose
- Use stress management techniques
- Eat moderately (and eat very little meat)
- Are involved with their families and their communities

One final interesting note about the Blue Zones: People who lived the longest were part of social networks that included other people who lived long lives — people whose healthy behaviors seemed to rub off on them.

The Well Living Lab

Current wellness research at Mayo Clinic includes a collaborative effort called the Well Living Lab with Delos, a company that specializes in health and wellness in the indoor environment. Delos focuses on transforming homes, offices, schools and other indoor environments into places that are designed to support health and wellness.

Research shows that most people spend 90 percent of their time indoors. With that in mind, together, Mayo Clinic and Delos are combining their expertise in health and building science to study indoor environments to determine how to better design and build healthier places to work, live, learn and play.

The Well Living Lab's research is informed by the WELL Building Standard, which includes seven pillars of wellness. The WELL Building Standard was developed by Delos and is administered by the International Well Building Institute.

The Well Living Lab simulates realistic living and working environments to monitor how well health-based interventions work. In the 7,500-square-foot lab, sensors measure how people react to changes in their environment. For example, you'll find a chair that buzzes when you've been sitting in it too long. Research shows that prolonged sitting is tied to poorer health, and even long hours at the gym do not offset the health risks of sitting too much. Interventions like the chair sensor illustrate one way that environments can be modified to encourage better health and wellness.

The Well Living Lab illustrates the goal of this entire book: that in order to truly improve your health and wellness, it's crucial to take an active role. Part of that responsibility involves looking around at your environment and giving some thought to basic changes that can help you become healthier — and happier.

Adapted from Buettner D. *The Blue Zones*. 2nd ed. Washington, D.C.: National Geographic; © 2012. Printed with permission.

Additional resources

Databases

Natural Medicines
1 Davis Square
Somerville, MA 02144
617-591-3300
https://naturalmedicines.therapeuticresearch.com

Organizations

**Academic Consortium
for Integrative Medicine & Health**
6728 Old McLean Village Drive
McLean, VA 22101
703-556-9222
www.imconsortium.org

**American Academy
of Medical Acupuncture**
2512 Artesia Blvd., Suite 200
Redondo Beach, CA 90278
310-379-8261
www.medicalacupuncture.org

American Academy of Osteopathy
3500 DePauw Blvd., Suite 1100
Indianapolis, IN 46268-1138
317-879-1881
www.academyofosteopathy.org

**American Association
of Acupuncture and Oriental Medicine**
P.O. Box 96503 #44114
Washington, DC 20090-6503
www.aaaomonline.org

**American Association
of Naturopathic Physicians**
818 18th St. NW, Suite 250
Washington, DC 20006
202-237-8150
www.naturopathic.org

American Botanical Council
P.O. Box 144345

Austin, TX 78714-4345
800-373-7105
http://abc.herbalgram.org

American Chiropractic Association
1701 Clarendon Blvd., Suite 200
Arlington, VA 22209
703-276-8800
www.acatoday.org

American Holistic Health Association
P.O. Box 17400
Anaheim, CA 92817-7400
714-779-6152
http://ahha.org

American Massage Therapy Association
500 Davis St., Suite 900
Evanston, IL 60201
877-905-0577
www.amtamassage.org

American Osteopathic Association
142 E. Ontario St.
Chicago, IL 60611-2864
888-626-9262
www.osteopathic.org

American Society of Clinical Hypnosis
140 N. Bloomingdale Road
Bloomingdale, IL 60108
630-980-4740
www.asch.net

**Association for Applied Psychophysiology
and Biofeedback**
10200 W. 44th Ave., Suite 304
Wheat Ridge, CO 80033
800-477-8892
www.aapb.org

ConsumerLab.com, LLC
333 Mamaroneck Ave.
White Plains, NY 10605
914-722-9149
www.consumerlab.com

**Food and Drug Administration,
Office of Dietary Supplement Programs**
5001 Campus Drive
College Park, MD 20740
888-723-3366
www.fda.gov/Food/DietarySupplements/default.htm

Healing Beyond Borders
445 Union Blvd., Suite 105
Lakewood, CO 80228
303-989-7982
www.healingbeyondborders.org

Mayo Clinic
www.MayoClinic.org

**National Association
for Holistic Aromatherapy**
P.O. Box 27871
Raleigh, NC 27611-7871
919-894-0298
www.naha.org

National Cancer Institute
BG 9609 MSC 9760
9609 Medical Center Drive
Bethesda, MD 20892-9760
800-422-6237
www.cancer.gov/about-cancer/treatment/cam

**National Center for Complementary and
Integrative Health**
9000 Rockville Pike
Bethesda, MD 20892
888-644-6226
https://nccih.nih.gov

National Center for Homeopathy
7918 Jones Branch Drive, Suite 300
McLean, VA 22102
703-506-7667
www.homeopathic.org

**Office of Cancer Complementary and
Alternative Medicine**
National Cancer Institute, NIH
9609 Medical Center Drive, Room 5-W-136
Rockville, MD 20850
240-276-6595
https://cam.cancer.gov

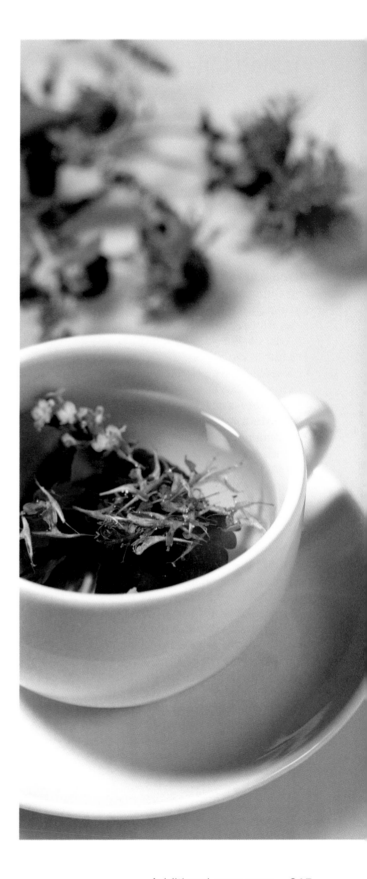

Visiting Mayo Clinic

Perhaps you were surprised to learn that doctors at Mayo Clinic incorporate practices such as massage and meditation into their care plans for patients. Or perhaps you're interested in the research Mayo Clinic is doing in the realm of integrative medicine. Maybe you have a condition that you feel might benefit from an integrative health care approach.

Regardless of your reason, if you're interested in being seen as a patient at Mayo Clinic, here are some things that might be helpful to know.

- You don't have to be referred to Mayo Clinic by a physician — but it helps.
- To make an appointment at one of our three locations, these are the numbers to call: Arizona, 800-446-2279; Florida, 904-953-0853; Minnesota, 507-538-3270.
- Your visit will usually begin with a complete physical examination by a general internal medicine physician.
- The doctor who performs your physical examination will refer you to a specialist if he or she feels a specialist can help.
- If you're interested in integrative therapies, express this interest to your Mayo physician. The form on page 204 may help you with talking points to discuss when you meet with your Mayo Clinic physician.
- You cannot make an appointment directly within the Mayo Clinic practice to receive treatments such as acupuncture, massage or meditation. You need to be referred for these services by a Mayo Clinic doctor.
- However, massage therapy and acupuncture are available to patients and their families when visiting the Mayo Clinic Healthy Living Program in Rochester, Minnesota. Make an appointment for a massage or for acupuncture, as well as spa services, by calling 507-293-2966 or by visiting *https://healthyliving.mayoclinic.org/rejuvenate-spa.php* for more information.

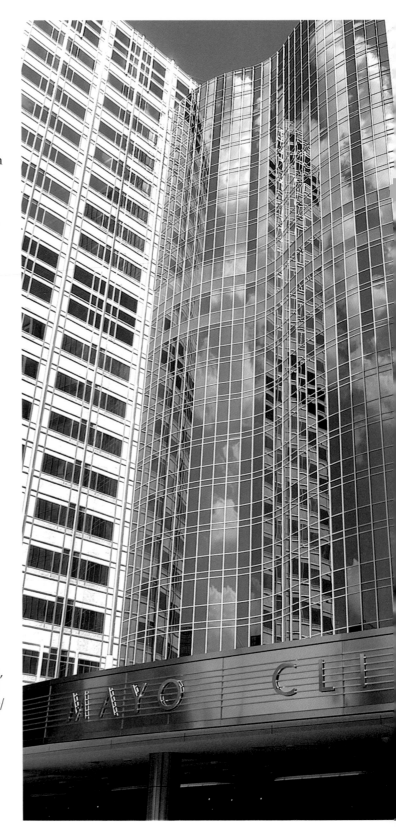

Index

Experts. Answers.

Mayo Clinic.

For complex medical conditions, answers can be hard to find. At Mayo Clinic, world-class experts work together, across specialties, to make sure you get exactly the care you need—care that's also covered by most insurance plans. It's a seamless approach to delivering complex care.

Make your appointment at **mayoclinic.org**.

MAYO CLINIC

Housecall

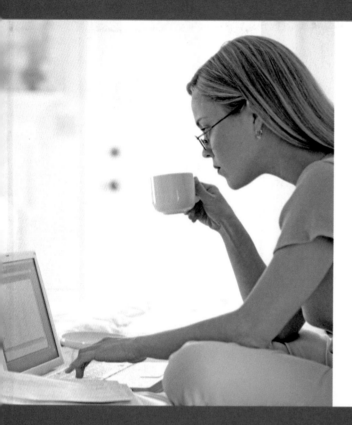

What our readers are saying ...

*"I depend on **Mayo Clinic Housecall** more than any other medical info that shows up on my computer. Thank you so very much."*

"Excellent newsletter. I always find something interesting to read and learn something new."

*"**Housecall** is a must read – keep up the good work!"*

*"I love **Housecall**. It is one of the most useful, trusted and beneficial things that come from the Internet."*

*"The **Housecall** is timely, interesting and invaluable in its information. Thanks much to Mayo Clinic for this resource!"*

"I enjoy getting the weekly newsletters. They provide me with friendly reminders, as well as information/ conditions I was not aware of."

Get the latest health information direct from Mayo Clinic ... Sign up today, it's FREE!

Mayo Clinic Housecall is a FREE weekly e-newsletter that offers the latest health information from the experts at Mayo Clinic. Stay up to date on topics that are current, interesting, and most of all important to your health and the health of your family.

What you get
- Weekly top story
- Additional healthy highlights
- Answers from the experts
- Quick access to trusted health tools
- Featured blogs
- Health tip of the week
- Special offers

Don't wait ... Join today!
MayoClinic.com/Housecall/Register

We're committed to helping you enjoy better health and get the most out of life every day. We hope you decide to become part of the Mayo Clinic family, where you can always count on receiving an interesting mix of health information from a trusted source.